Collateral Damage

When Caregivers No Longer Care

Adonis & Abbey Publishers Ltd
24 Old Queen Street, London SW1H 9HP United Kingdom
Website: http://www.adonis-abbey.com
E-mail Address: editor@adonis-abbey.com

Website: http://www.adonis-abbey.com
E-mail Address: editor@adonis-abbey.com

Nigeria:
No. 39 Jimmy Carter Street, Suites C3 – C6 J-Plus Plaza Asokoro, Abuja, Nigeria
Tel: +234 (0) 7058078841/08052035034

British Library Cataloguing-in-Publication Data
A catalogue record for this book is available from the British Library

ISBN: 9781913976187

Photo of "Man Hand in Protective Gloves Holding Red Heart on Blue" on book cover is from ©towfiqu barbhuiya via canva.com. The sky background is a photo taken by a friend of Greg Noack; used with permission.

Collateral Damage

When Caregivers No Longer Care

Greg Noack

Adonis & Abbey
Publishers Ltd

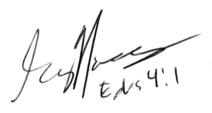

Table of Contents

Prologue

I had the privilege and honor to have my book ***My Invisible Disability*** published in February 2006. I never knew the effort involved and the length of time required in getting a book published.

The book took me five years to piece together and is based on journals I wrote while recovering and rehabilitating from a severe traumatic brain injury that I suffered in the fall of 1996.

It took another five years looking for and finding a publisher. My book was unsolicited and written by me, an unknown author. So, after receiving numerous rejection letters from publishers in North America, I decided to send a query letter to a publishing house in London, England, called Adonis & Abbey Publishers.

Adonis & Abbey Publishers showed interest and wanted a sample chapter. From this, the publishing firm assisted in getting my book printed, published and available to all on the World Wide Web.

I continued with my writing, in note pads or typing random thoughts on a computer, since 2001 while working full time in health care. Being a person with a brain injury, I suffer from fatigue, a symptom of my brain injury, and have been unable to really focus on writing due to working full time. Before my brain injury, I had the ability to do both, work and write, but now I have to prioritize.

The random thoughts I jotted down or typed focused on my experiences working in health care over the years and brought me back to memories of my life right after discharge from rehab. I decided to write more about my experiences with health care and the facilities that provide care because of my father's treatment during his battle with lung cancer.

The capital white letter H with the blue background symbolizes a hospital in Canada and I was first introduced to a hospital on July 2, 1972, when I came into this world. At that time, the H stood for happy, as my parents had their third of four children.

You will read about my experiences with hospitals, first from being a patient going through a year of recovery and rehabilitation as a result of a traumatic brain injury caused by a violent assault, to becoming a clinician; I have worked in the field of neuro rehabilitation and research in some capacity the past twenty years; and lastly as an advocating family member, supporting and observing my father fight the horrible disease of lung cancer.

These three personas – patient, clinician, and advocate – that I became have one trait in common, vulnerability. As you will read, accepting our vulnerability will allow us to deal with our own expectations and perceptions of not only hospitals but those who provide care. Sharing my experiences, good and bad, I hope will change what is expected from health care and the clinicians and staff that work in this industry and how they are perceived.

Dedication

This is for you dad, you never wanted to rock the boat, but I am going to try to make waves to change things down here. Love you.

Foreword

"The hurt is how we know
We are alive & awake;
It clears us for all the exquisite,
Excruciating enormities to come.
We are pierced new by the turning
Forward.
. . .
What we carry means we survive,
It is what survives us.
We have survived us.
Where once we were alone,
Now we are beside ourselves."
Amanda Gorman. "Good Grief."Call Us What We Carry, Viking/Penguin Random House, 2021. (Lines 14-19, 31-35)

Greg Noack's new book exemplifies this notion of turning forward, purposely and authentically calling into the light "what we carry" in order to improve our eyesight. The genesis of this book is the author's desire to share what he carries in order to summon us back to a time when we were truly connected to our purpose as clinicians, before perhaps routine, burnout and apathy drained us of our passion and compassion. Leveraging his lived experience as both a patient surviving a traumatic beating, navigating the long term effects of a traumatic brain injury, and his work as a rehabilitation clinician, Greg's story lays bare possibility and humanness in the midst of loss, grief and pain.

Greg's life and writing demonstrates the power of traversing through adversity into new ways of being and doing. He challenges us to aspire to higher levels of self-awareness, to be our best selves with others, not just to help ourselves but to trust, listen and learn from the wisdom of those we care for. It is often not the professional therapeutic interventions that make a difference. Rather it is the smallest of our words and actions that create new pathways to healing or destroy hope and marginalize those who need us at this most difficult time in their lives.

As we emerge from the isolation and suffering of the recent COVID pandemic, hibernating from our own humanity (Gorman, 2021), Greg's story takes on a new resonance. Compassion for our patients AND our colleagues need be our compass, the true north that brings us to our work, our sense of purpose and unique contribution. Through Greg's experiences, we see the power of insight and compassion that will lead us back to an understanding of who we are as human beings, to refresh our basic human qualities of generosity, compassion, deep listening. We each are what we carry. What we carry means we survive. By turning forward with compassion to what survives us, I trust we will not only survive but thrive!

Joy Richards, PhD, RN, FAAN
Vice-President University Health Network (UHN),
Health Education Development & Executive-in-Residence Michener Institute UHN
Toronto, Canada

"As a prisoner of the Lord, then, I urge you to live a life worthy of the calling you have received."

Ephesians 4:1 (New International Version)[1]

Book One

HEAD INJURY & HOPE

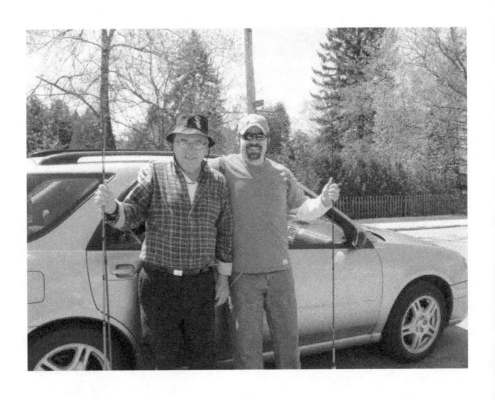

CHAPTER ONE

Reborn

Other than my birth, which of course I do not remember, I had minimal experiences with a hospital in my early years. My brother Scott, who was two years older, struck me with a golf club when I was five years old. The strike was accidental as I was his caddy and was standing too close when he swung his club. I always was attached to my big brother when I was young, too close in this case.

I also was struck playing schoolyard cricket during recess when I was 11 years old. My friend on the opposing team took a second swing at the rubber ball we used and I, of course, was on the receiving end of the swing as I caught the ball.

The broken hockey sticks we used as our cricket bats sliced beneath my right eye, shattering my cheekbone and left a laceration almost to my ear resulting in 50 stitches. I do remember bits of this experience: my grade seven teacher cursing in terror when he came to help and at the hospital in my hometown of Sault Ste. Marie, Ontario when my family doctor stated,

"We have to get someone else to do this." A surgeon flew in from Toronto and the five-hour wait was worth it as you can barely see the scar from such a vicious strike.

In both cases, I am very grateful I did not lose an eye. I also was too young to realize how fortunate I was to be in Canada with access to universal health care; the expenses and my surgery were covered by our government. After coming close to losing an eye the second time, I did not have any other experience with hospitals for the next 13 years. When I did, it changed me forever.

"What time is it, man?"

"I don't know. We have been here all night and I am still pretty messed up."

The party was starting to die down as it was approaching four thirty in the morning.

All that remained were the tenants of the party residence, someone who was raiding the fridge and two others who at the moment were trying to figure out when they arrived and how they ended up so inebriated.

"Let's get Jimmy and get out of here."

Jimmy was the least affected by substances used, alcohol and pot that is so popular out west in British Columbia and was very popular at this party.

"Hey, guys. Ready to head?" Jimmy said, approaching his scrunched up and lifeless friends, who shared a third of a couch, as the owners were passed out on the other two thirds.

"Yeah, there is a coffee shop down the road that I wouldn't mind hitting. Shit I'm hungry."

"Me too."

The three left, leaving the dank apartment that now showed the good times held by the fifty to a hundred people who drank and smoked the previous night away.

"F—k it is foggy out."

The three staggered and approached the bridge part of the Gorge Road.

"I got to take a piss. Wait a minute."

The bridge was above a heavily wooded trail that was used for such leisurely activities as biking or hiking. The road allowed you entrance to the trail on both ends of the bridge by walking down about ten stairs. Jimmy and his partner stood and waited as their friend walked down the stairs and got lost in the trees to urinate. He could have urinated on the street with the fog as heavy as it was but, in his state of mind, he still wanted to find some privacy.

"Hey, Jimmy, look at this guy! Why is he crossing the street? Does he think we're going to hurt him?"

"Just leave him be."

"I'm gonna give him a reason for crossing the f--king street."

Jimmy did not like how this was shaping up so he became part of the situation and hopefully could contain the escalation.

"Hey, man; wait for me," Jimmy spoke as his friend increased his pace while crossing the street to put the scare into the passer-by.

"Hey, asshole!"

Jimmy interrupted his suddenly angry friend before he continued and politely said, "Yeah, we were wondering if you have any change for a coffee?"

The young man nervously removed one of the gloves he was wearing and reached into his pocket. Before he raised his hand out of his jean's pocket, a thud similar to a baseball bat hitting a melon broke the silent morning. With the sound came debris in the form of the toque the young man was wearing, blood and splinters from the explosion of wood on skull.

"What the hell?" Jimmy asked as the jittery person, who was obliging in giving him change, fell forward into his chest and then slowly down his body as Jimmy took baby steps back to see what had happened.

When Jimmy did step back and lifted his eyes from the fallen stranger, he noticed his friend who had gone to urinate standing a body distance away holding what looked like a two by four chunk of wood. He had grabbed wood from down on the trail where the city was constructing a fence.

"Why did you do that?" Jimmy asked with great despair in his voice.

There was no response and before Jimmy took another gasp of air his two friends were on the now unconscious victim and proceeded to taunt his lifeless body. These taunts were starting to escalate and led to kicks to his head.

"Stop it. You're going to kill him!"

"Shut the f—k up, Jimmy."

Stomps were also included in the kicks as the two turned their scared prey's body over and proceeded to do the same. Jimmy could not take it any longer and ran off into the fog.

"Victoria Police."

"Yeah, ah," Jimmy's voice was affected by running and what he had just witnessed.

"There is a guy under the Gorge Road Bridge in rough shape."

"And you are."

Before the dispatcher could ask anything else, the line went dead. The dispatcher could not trace anything because Jimmy called from a payphone. Due to the shortness and abruptness of the call, the dispatcher did not send anyone to look into the seriousness of the hang-up. Back on the bridge, one of the partygoers was on his knees, straddling the unexpected party and attempting to strangle out any life that was left in him.

"Okay, man. Let's go. A car is coming."

The strangler got up and once up grabbed his victim by the shirt, lifting his limp body up, about two feet off the ground, and spoke, "F--ker, no more crossing the street for you."

He shoved him to the ground and ran off into the fog that now hid what he had done. The innocent person, who crossed the street for this very reason, to avoid confrontation, lay there for approximately one hour until someone who was going in for his or her early shift at work discovered him. His eyes in his unconscious body were still open but he could not see.

This is the best for him, for me. Not remembering or knowing eliminated any fear I would have of living the remainder of my life in this sometimes dark and evil place. Also now believing that this place is not my last stop helps as well. Jimmy tried to help, but his call went unanswered. He did see that night and now has to deal with what he saw. I feel for him and pray that he knows there is better.

"I once was lost, but now I am found; was blind, but now I see."
'Amazing Grace' – John Newton (Olney Hymns, 1779)

Starting path - November 30th, 1996

My mother, Diane, was meeting with Gail, the social worker, at the acute care hospital. This was an important meeting in determining the next step in my recovery from the catastrophic brain injury I suffered from an assault almost three weeks earlier. Two of these weeks plus a day were spent in a coma.

My mom was still in shock as, minutes earlier, Gail had met with me to discuss how things were going. My mom and my roommate Allison had difficulty sitting me up at my bedside without me falling over let alone me concentrating on questions about how things were going with my recovery from a traumatic event causing brain damage.

I succeeded sitting up and nodding at Gail. To this day, I still do not remember this meeting but someone up above knew it was time for me to leave the acute care hospital and move on. This forgotten meeting was instrumental in showing Gail I was making progress and that moving on to a rehabilitation facility that provided intensive therapy was a viable option.

Health care begins in acute care and then through time your path begins. For me the path would move from acute care onto intensive rehabilitation.

"Greg seems well and has made gains, especially considering he just woke under a week ago," Gail spoke.

"Yes."

My mom's one-word response was caused by the miracle that she had just witnessed minutes earlier. She did an amazing job of hiding her emotions.

"So, Diane, the Gorge Road Rehabilitation Hospital has a bed opening up in a few days. So, if Greg continues to progress, we will transfer him there," Gail stated, handing my mother an admissions folder with information on the Gorge and what my stay would encompass.

"Greg's apartment is on Gorge road," my mother replied while shuffling through the folder just given to her.

As my mom read the information, she became excited as she knew this was the best path for me to take. She knew that if I went somewhere else, a place where rehabilitation was intensive, I may not continue to progress and have less a chance at regaining my independence.

"That is great. It is good that you are close, making visits less of a hassle."

Gail was a compassionate social worker, who was concerned about not only me but also the effects my ordeal had on my mother.

"Just a couple things, Diane," Gail said, turning the pages of my medical chart that had my progress documented by the various professionals who had provided my care.

My mother was nervous as she did not want to 'mess up' this great opportunity.

"Would you say Greg has gotten more alert? I know it is just under a week since his awakening and he needs his rest, but do you feel he could handle a daily therapy schedule?"

"Think so. Cannot really say because of the unknown, but God willing."

"Diane, I asked because the Gorge is a transitional hospital, about a 4-8 week stay, meaning if he does not settle or progress, we have to think of the options after that. Where would Greg live after this time?"

Before Gail could say any of the options, my mom blurted out, "With me."

"Excellent," Gail said while writing.

Gail knew that there was a chance I could be a 'handful' but the healthcare team at the Gorge would get the 'ball rolling' in helping my mother with this transition if need be.

"Is Greg continent?" Gail asked.

This was a big question that could cause my admission to the Gorge difficult as knowing when I had to go to the bathroom would make my admission more appropriate.

"He is still in diapers (pull-up disposable briefs) but knows when he needs to go."

My mother is a devout Christian who just lied but understood the consequences of telling the truth.

"Good. So December third we will send Greg to the Gorge. We just have some forms to fill out."

"Thank you, Gail. I am so happy for my son," my mom stated, becoming emotional. "I know, Diane. I know."

The chart, I am sure, stated to Gail my mother had lied about my continence, but Gail gave me a chance. I also did not know the pressures she was under at freeing up a bed for the next person to come in. The pressure to free up beds in acute care was similar to my recovery from brain injury, unknown and unpredictable, as you never knew when a need for beds would occur. Who can predict events that cause trauma and the need for a bed and emergency services? There also may have been pressure on the Gorge to fill their bed as well. Beds need to be filled for funding for rehabilitation programs from the government, and overlooking my incontinence may have helped both facilities.

I did not mind, neither did my mother, even though she changed my disposable briefs and kept our secret and lie from the staff at the Gorge, until I became continent. We can both live with this lie.

Phase 2

It was two months after my assault and I was beginning out-patient therapy. Out-patient meaning I was out of the hospital. I did not realize the importance of the word 'out' as it applied to patient therapy as some did not progress as far as I did in their rehabilitation and remained in the hospital and then were discharged to another destination other than their own home. I did not have to move in with my mother or need the level of assistance provided by a long term care facility.

My therapy sessions consisted of physiotherapy (PT) on Tuesday and Thursday afternoons for one hour, and occupational therapy (OT) Monday and Wednesday mornings for an hour. I would meet John, the social worker from the Gorge, once a month as well. Not as intensive rehabilitation as the previous month when I was an inpatient as I was progressing and needed less therapy. Also, my time was up and others needed the opportunity for intense rehabilitation.

Allison, my roommate who became my girlfriend, came in with me for my first OT session. It was very convenient that my therapy was located at the same hospital where I was a patient. Being familiar to me was important and seeing my friends that gained through my rehabilitation daily was a bonus. Only having to walk ten minutes to the front door would give me my independence once I got comfortable going alone. Bob also lived there so seeing him was the greatest bonus of all.

Bob was an amazing man, the first person I opened up to and communicated with when I first arrived at the rehabilitation hospital as an inpatient. He was seventy-eight years old and was full of such knowledge. I dedicated my first book, ***My Invisible Disability*** (Adonis & Abbey Publishers, 2006) which entails my two months of recovery and inpatient rehabilitation, to him. How he responded to his botched surgery and the situation he was put into from it was one of many perspectives I would gain from him.

I was quite fatigued from an exciting weekend – my first weekend – knowing I would not have to return to the hospital and adjust to life at home. Even though I was away from home for only two months, it felt like I was getting off the plane in Vancouver again, starting over, and unlike when I first arrived in British Columbia, employment was now the least of my concerns. Adapting to what deficits my brain injury would leave me set in.

I also had a restless sleep, which added to my already present fatigue. My restlessness was caused by nerves brought on by my therapy and whether or not I would get along with my new therapists. Just doing therapy set off a deep anger that I started to control but was festering. I was doing therapy as a result of an assault that I could not remember, and this was at the heart of my anger.

Therapy from the beginning frightened me. I wanted to get better but was afraid to find out my limitations caused by my brain injury. I was scared of reaching my plateau in recovery, not being able to recover any further. I was grateful to walk again and felt great physically, other than exhaustion, but was concerned about the mental aspect of my rehabilitation. I did not really know what this entailed. Having such insight was a positive thing, and I wanted to know and become aware of my limitations, no matter how angry it made me feel.

I accepted the unknown of brain injury quite early and learned that this acceptance would allow me to rely on others, for the time being.

Allison and I introduced who we were to the front desk.

"Hello, Greg. I'm Edith."

"Hello, this is my girlfriend Allison."

Edith was my occupational therapist who would continue on with therapy that focused on my cognitive abilities. We followed Edith into the room where Paula, my occupational therapist when I was an inpatient, had tested my eyes. We sat in front of one of the many computers.

"Okay, Greg. We are going to do several activities and tests on the computer. I will now show you how to turn on the computer and get to the menu of games that you will be doing."

Edith explained how to turn the computer 'off' and 'on' and the steps required getting to the games menu. When she was finished, I then had to do it, telling her the steps involved. I was correct and looked at Allison seated to the right of me, giving her a smirk and rolling my eyes. I found the beginning of our session comical, not realizing Edith was testing my immediate memory. The simple act of following instructions to turning a computer on and finding a game was a gauge for sequencing and memory. I passed this test and found it unusual, ignorant of the fact others that had suffered a brain injury may have not made it past this first step.

Once I was at the 'games' menu, Edith made me highlight a game called 'Arrows'. She explained the instructions to the game. I then had to recite what she had said, explaining the game to her.

"Greg, we will start at level three. There are ten levels."

I then proceeded with the game as Edith stepped out for a minute. 'Arrows' was a game where I had to find arrows located on a grid. I would type in coordinates on the x-axis and y-axis. It was a process of elimination similar to the game 'You sunk my battleship'. Edith returned and I had successfully found all the arrows.

"Well done, Greg. We will try again at five."

"I'm not coming back at five o'clock," I abruptly answered as I stared at Allison with a look of, 'Yeah right, you are crazy, lady, to think I am coming back at five at night.'

"Level five, Greg," Edith replied while writing in her note pad.

"Ohhh," I responded as Allison and I started to chuckle, getting the giggles.

It was funny but sad. This was a sign of a limitation brought on by my brain injury. Taking things literally and applying only one meaning to something that had more than one. I continued on with 'Arrows', completing level five with no mistakes, and wanted to try it at seven, level seven.

CHAPTER TWO

Ignorance Begins

I met with my financial assistance worker (FAW) two weeks after I had been discharged from being an inpatient at the Gorge. I was given information by the neurologist who tended to me, stating that I would not be capable of working for the next year, possibly two. With the disability of brain injury, doctors need time to see how you will recover with two years set as a time frame. At the end of two years, whatever deficits left from my brain injury would more than likely be everlasting.

I would speak to other professionals who stated that, in fifteen years, there was a chance of noticing recovery from something I had lost. Time regarding recovery from neurological trauma is not found in textbooks because every brain is different and reacts differently to trauma or disease. I concentrated on the latter and that maybe down the road I would regain my energy, even though possibly unrealistic, why not think positively?

Mom, Allison, and I drove to the social assistance office, not knowing what to expect, not compassion. The 'system', which I did not ever want to be dependent of, now needed to support me. When I needed them the most, they did not help. The assistance I had received so far was minimal. It all began two days after my assault.

The government worker assigned to me, upon hearing what had happened to me from my mother, came into the hospital to see that I was comatose to verify my mother's story. Hearing this made me sick as the taxes I paid ever since I worked from the age of sixteen, or when I purchased something, went towards a system meant to help and support persons in situations like mine.

Instead of assisting and giving me what I was entitled to, it seemed like the aim of the worker on my case was to withhold and give the least assistance possible. When I was hospitalized, I received three hundred dollars along with a paltry eight dollars for hygienic items and any other expenses. They even considered the hospital my home. Just receiving this was difficult but the provincial government, the 'system', finally gave in. I assume my mother needing a place to stay and Allison having to find a new place to live because her roommate was nearly beaten to death on

Victoria's 'safe' streets swayed their decision.

The three of us got out of the car, with me holding my mom for support as I walked. Once in the office, my FAW introduced himself and offered the three of us seats in front of his desk. Right from the beginning, I despised him. He did not care. I could not help but paint him with such a brush as he gave my loved ones no help. I now was going to experience this first-hand as well.

"Greg, what we are going to do is place you in the unemployable section of financial assistance."

The province had three categories, each having different monetary amounts. The other two were employable and disability. I applied for disability, federally, and made the assumption this was the same as the provincial category. My FAW reinforced such by not placing me in that section or giving me the proper forms to apply.

"We will put you in the employable section when your doctor determines when you can work again."

The assistance I would now receive would continue to cover my rent plus two hundred dollars for living expenses. Not a lot, considering my phone bill alone was well over one hundred dollars and along with heat and other bills; I had no idea how I would get by. I even had fifty dollars a month to pay back on my student loan for my failed year at university five years earlier. I still had to pay for that mistake with the government not being lenient no matter what my situation was.

My FAW then leaned forward so that only I could hear, "Greg, you look fine. If you ever feel like working, go ahead and work."

I hesitantly smiled. I did not know what to make of what he said. I viewed it as a compliment but also was perplexed. At the beginning of the meeting, I handed him information from a doctor that treated me stating I may not be employable for up to two years with the possibility of never working again.

Health care professionals viewed what happened to me as disabling. How come my FAW did not? He just looked at my appearance and made his judgment. He did not see me before my assault and was not aware of me losing fifty pounds in fifteen days. He was not there when I was in disposable briefs as I did not have the ability to go to the bathroom without assistance. He did not see me having to relearn how to walk, laugh, and cry. He was ignorant of me and brain injuries. I was ignorant of my rights and what I was entitled to because of my situation and disability. How was I supposed to know? This was my FAW's job and, being ignorant of the system, I assumed he was doing a good job and being helpful.

We got up and he walked us to the front door. I had to provide him with a medical report every three months to determine my assistance. As we left he spoke to me, "Remember what I said."

When mom, Allison and I began the drive home, mom asked, "Remember what, Greg?"

"Nothing."

I looked out the window with tired eyes, knowing I had to get a job.

Reluctance

I had a meeting with John, my social worker, and Brenda, a lady who had worked with me previously in occupational therapy when I was an inpatient. The two wanted to hear how my first week of outpatient therapy was going and how I was adjusting to the 'outside world'. I went into the meeting with what my financial assistance worker stated. I was flustered and panic-stricken, fearing I would have to resort back to mopping floors to get by.

"How are things going in therapy, Greg?" John asked.

Both he and Brenda had pen and paper waiting to write down my responses. Something I had grown accustomed to. It seemed every move I made, or whatever I stated, was being observed and analyzed, from rehab to the government. I was developing a 'big brother' complex.

"Fine, I like my therapists."

"How are you doing at home?"

"Good. I am worried though. I have to start looking for work to pay the bills and support myself."

After my answer, John and Brenda looked at each other and John then spoke in paused amazement, "Greg, you need a bit of time yet to recover and rest."

"Yes, Greg. Thinking of work should be the farthest from your mind. You need to rest and deal with your trauma," Brenda added.

"But how am I supposed to get by?"

The two were probably used to this question, especially dealing with the bureaucracy of the government for financial assistance and the system's lack of compassion for not only persons with brain injury but also those with mental issues that are not always visible and difficult to prove.

"I know, Greg, that you are not being compensated properly for what you have been through. No monetary amount is enough for what you went through. You have to use your support system, both financially and mentally."

After John had spoken, whatever independence I had gained by moving out west evaporated. I now had to rely on a system that viewed me as everyone else, just an abuser of society's giving. Worse than this, I would have to rely on my mother and loved ones for support financially as well, something I never wanted to do. I had no other choice which started to light the fuse of my already growing anger. I now could not work to avoid such dependence.

Brenda then spoke to John, "You know who would be good for Greg, Robin."

"Yes. I will see if I could swing it with funding from the hospital. Greg, what we are going to do is try and set up some sessions with Robin, a psychologist, who is excellent dealing with people with your problems," John said.

"Okay," I replied.

"Hopefully by the end of the week, we will have something lined up."

"Thank you."

"You are welcome," John and Brenda responded.

"Greg, Brenda and I will meet with you again in a month's time say mid-February, to see how things are progressing. I will contact you later in the week regarding sessions with Robin."

"Thanks you two. Good-bye."

"Bye, Greg."

As I left John's office, I overheard the two muttering about what they had just heard and how I was concerned about finding employment this soon in my recovery. They were there, however, to see what I went through while the 'system' was not. The signals I received from them and the government confused me. What was I going to do?

Different Route

My mother and I entered extended care (aka long term care/LTC) of the rehabilitation hospital to see Bob.

"When I leave to go back to Powell River, you make sure you come to see Bob at least once a week," mom said.

"I definitely will."

Powell River, British Columbia was a small community on the mainland approximately five hours from Victoria. This is where my stepfather Brian lived and where my mother could finally get started with her married life. It was delayed by three months by what had happened to me.

As we turned the corner of the basement floor of extended care, I was shocked and saddened. All I saw was shriveled up human life in complex wheelchairs or scooters. Some of them staring off into space, with others laughing at their own jokes or laughing because that was what their brains had told them to do. The 'conveyer belt', known as health care, that I was on, ended here sometimes in a warehouse of forgotten souls. I was fortunate to go on an opposite path at the end of the belt.

Mother and I looked at each other, our faces flat with expression from what we were seeing. Mine was flat purposely this time, not caused by my brain injury.

"Bob should not be here, mom."

"I know, Greg. I know."

The only reason he was, was because the health care road stopped for him. The doctors and therapists felt he had reached a plateau in his recovery and once reached, extended care became his home. Bob's caring heart also played a part because he was capable of living back at home with assistance and I am sure his family wanted him to, but he did not want to be a burden on anyone. He also was determined to walk again and viewed extended care as temporary.

We entered Bob's room and he was in his wheelchair in front of his window staring outside. His three roommates were incapable of carrying on a conversation due to their illnesses.

"Hey pal," I said.

"Greg and Dianne, how are you?"

I gave Bob a hug followed by mom giving a hug and a kiss.

"I am fine."

"Good," mom added.

"Bob, we got to get you out of here. I will take you home with me," mom said jokingly but with a serious undertone in her voice, shaken from what she was observing.

"Do not worry, you two. I will be okay. Do you want to go to the cafeteria and have a coffee or tea?"

"Sure," we both replied.

While we walked through Bob's new home, I whispered to mom, "We got to get him out of here." Mom nodded in agreement.

I was extremely agitated at how the hospital had given up on him. Once in extended care, your therapy was gradually stopped. How could they do this to Bob? I know his age did not help him. We heard several groans as we made our way to the cafeteria and Bob replied, "I think that is my roommate Ronny and that other is my roommate Joey."

I did not know whether to laugh or cry.

We sat down for our tea and coffee, with mom buying Bob a large oatmeal cookie for later. I looked around my surroundings as we settled in at our table. I was overwhelmed, from a young man whose body shook uncontrollable from Parkinson's disease to a middle-aged woman who communicated by a thumb up and print out from an electronic device attached to her wheelchair. Bob enlightened us with all their stories and an ache developed in my chest. It did not surprise me that Bob knew such horrific information as he had found out mine and now was finding out theirs to give help. This also showed me tragedy had no set demographic.

"Bob, why do you have to stay here?" I was starting to lose control of my emotions.

"You have to be patient, Greg. I am going to go to physiotherapy and acupuncture of my own accord. I will walk out this place when it is time for me to leave," coming from a seventy-nine-year-old man who had triple by-pass surgery resulting in his inability to walk.

"I know you will, I know you will."

"You sure will," mom added.

After coffee, we walked back beside Bob to his room. Bob told a couple of inhabitants to smile and keep smiling, tapping them on the knees as we moved by. Once in his room, Bob situated himself by the window with the big oatmeal cookie mom had bought him on his lap. We said our goodbyes and I mentioned I would come for a visit early next week. While leaving, I turned back as Bob began to unravel the plastic from his cookie and staring outside. This brilliant and intelligent man had no one to share his insights and knowledge with.

"How friggin' sad," I said to mom.

"I know. This is bullshit," mom replied with an unusual curse.

"You make sure you come and see him once a week."

"I will, mom. I will."

Even though I became exhausted from fatigue caused as much by physical activity as emotions, I would see Bob every day. He was there for me and I was going to be there for him. Out-patient therapy took place and was located right down the hall. The cafeteria was the fork in the road.

CHAPTER THREE

Battles

My outpatient physiotherapist Beth noticed the footwear I was wearing in our first session. I had all white, cheaper shoes/'sneakers' that lacked any arch support that my foot needed. They were brand new as my mother purchased them for me due to all I had at that moment to wear was work shoes/boots for my janitorial job, and hikers that I wore during my off time. I did not have proper footwear for a physiotherapy treatment session.

I had contacted Social Services, telling them of my 'shoe' situation and provided them with a letter Beth had written regarding my need for proper footwear. Surprisingly, they stated they would assist me in covering the cost. I would have to go out and get quotes for the type of shoes I needed and provide them with the necessary information.

I would walk to a variety of stores and this would add to my fatigue. I was of the mindset of pushing myself to build up my tolerance/endurance, even though I was forewarned by Beth, and numerous health care professionals of 'over doing it' and the importance of rest. I never would use the transit system as I was not yet comfortable with confronting a busload of strangers.

After two weeks of an exhausting search, I found shoes that met my needs, even though a lower cost was over one hundred dollars. The government was flipping the bill, but I still looked for the best bargain.

"Hello, Social Services."

"Hello. I am calling regarding funding for new shoes."

"Your SIN number (social insurance number)."

Whenever I called Social Services, I was never asked my name or to divulge any other information until they had heard that nine-digit number. I never used it prior to my ordeal but displayed good memory and recall as I listed those nine digits with great ease. Repetition is an excellent memory strategy.

"Okay, Gregory. I have your file and it states we would provide you with funding for shoes."

"Great. The ones I need cost one hundred and twenty dollars."

I just finished speaking when I was abruptly snapped at.

"We do not give that much for running shoes."

"But I was told to go and get quotes, and that is the lowest quote that met my needs."

"We only give fifty dollars towards shoes. That is it."

I felt her anger escalating by the tone of her voice.

"But I went to several stores."

"So, just fifty dollars. That is it!" she snapped again.

I was becoming emotional and short of breath. I was tired of this treatment. This treatment never changed, from my financial assistance worker on my casefile to any person who would answer the phone when I called. They continually accumulated information on my situation and, with this knowledge, would come greater ignorance towards me. I had enough.

"Yes, what is your name?" I asked in a voice becoming muffled from near weeping.

"Mrs. Smith. Do you want me to spell it?"

Her rudeness was beyond what I could take.

"No." And with my answer I hung up the phone, ending our conversation.

Right after I had hung up, I picked up the phone again and called my mother.

"Hello," she answered after the second ring.

"Ma…" I began to cry.

"What son?" my mother was panic-stricken, thinking of the worse.

I composed myself with some deep breaths.

"Why are they like this to me? I did not mean for this to happen."

"Who?" mom asked, growing anxious for my response.

"Social Services."

"What happened?"

"I called about my shoes but the lady was so rude, stating they only give fifty bucks towards shoes. This was the first time they have told me this. I would have never gone to all those shoe places if I had known this."

"I know they should have," mom was getting frustrated with my mistreatment.

"Did you get the person's name?" she inquired.

"Yes. Mrs. Smith. When I asked for it, she wondered if she had to spell it for me. She made me feel like an invalid."

"Okay, I have the number to Social Services. I will take care of it. When I come to see you in a couple of days, we will head up to the office and get the money for your shoes. I will let you go and call you back. Bye, Greg. Love you."

"Love you too."

My mom did not want to let herself cool down; she wanted to get to the bottom of this. And she did. We went up to the office two days later and received a check to cover the cost of my shoes. I met Mrs. Smith and, as she handed me the check, she stated, "Now we are not that difficult to deal with, are we?"

I did not respond to the statement and looked to my mother, who shook her head in disgust. She would later reveal to me how Mrs. Smith, in her conversation with her, had said I misinterpreted what she had said and that I overreacted. Mrs. Smith blamed my brain injury as an excuse for her disgusting behavior. My mother was biased towards me but she knew Mrs. Smith's treatment of me was real and she was starting to get sick of it.

A Mother's Perspective

I will begin our story (my son's and mine). On November 10, 1996 when, as a mother, my worst fear became a reality. I received a telephone call from my son's roommate in Victoria; Greg had been brutally attacked while walking home from work and left unconscious on Gorge Road.

There were no signs of a struggle, no marks on his hands; all the blows were to his head. The police said it was evident he had been struck from behind and had no chance to defend himself.

To this date, the police have not identified Greg's assailants. A reward has been offered by 'Crime stoppers' and there has been little response.

With that first blow, Greg's life changed forever. Greg became a "Victim". He would find out in months to come that he would be victimized by the system as well.

Brian (Greg's stepfather) and I left Powell River on that very day that the call came and rushed to Victoria General Hospital. Greg had been admitted to the intensive care unit in critical condition. He had suffered severe trauma to his head.

When I entered his room, I couldn't even recognize my son; his face was so swollen and bruised and tears mixed with blood trickled from the corners of his eyes. Machines surrounded his bed with wires connected to his skull, chest and arms; these wires were everywhere. I couldn't understand how anyone could treat a fellow human being with such cruelty.

Greg had lapsed into a coma. Fifteen days past and with each day a new concern. Greg's father flew out to see him and then had to return to Ontario. Greg's condition deteriorated. I continued to pray that Greg wouldn't leave this earth before me, parents die first.

The social worker at Victoria General met with Greg's roommate and me to prepare us for the worst. She was very compassionate and suggested we prepare for both case scenarios, recovery with only some lingering problems or the possibility that Greg may not pull through. I chose to focus on the positive that Greg was going to come back to us. I wanted that feeling projected in his room.

Greg's brother Scott and sisters, Kim and Melissa, flew to Victoria because we all wanted to be together in case Greg lost this battle. We watched his body stiffen, in medical terms 'posture'. His arms curled tightly into his chest, they were so rigid that you couldn't pull them free. The longer he remained in the coma, the longer it would take to recover. His body shook with seizures; there was constant noise from the machines. His heart rate was erratic. A rod was inserted into his skull to monitor the swelling of his brain.

There was always the fear that pneumonia would set in. The neurosurgeons could not give me any definitive answers to my questions because the recovery from brain injury follows no predictable pattern.

God answered the prayers of many. I entered his room after taking a few hours of much needed rest and was greeted with "Hi, mom."

I couldn't stop crying, I have never felt such joy.

Greg was an infant again. He wore a diaper (I kept thinking how modest he used to be). He couldn't stand, sit up, hold his head up, feed himself or swallow. Any noise disturbed him. After Greg had come out of the coma, his brother and sisters returned to Ontario. Greg's roommate Allison and I rarely left Greg's side. Without supervision, he would try to disconnect the tubes that were giving him his nourishment so the nurses would have to tie him to his bed.

By the first week of December, he had made enough progress that a decision was made to send Greg to the Gorge Road Rehabilitation Hospital. This was the beginning of yet another long battle. The staff was excellent; they provided a cot so I could stay in Greg's room at night. Greg's roommate and I alternated with one person in the morning and afternoon, the other in the evening and night. Greg began the long difficult process of learning everything again. He had to learn how to bathe himself, comb his hair, hold a spoon, sit, stand, walk, read, and the list goes on. His life became continuous therapy.

Greg was able to leave the rehab hospital after one month as an inpatient. We were all very encouraged and were under the misconception that Greg's struggles would become less difficult. This hasn't been the case.

As you are aware, from the information given in this letter, Greg was not injured at his place of employment so workers compensation is not a factor. He was not in a vehicular accident so there is no provincial insurance. Greg is a 'Victim of a Crime'. He doesn't fit in any category.

At the present time, Greg cannot be gainfully employed. He suffers from seizures, which are controlled by medication and he is unable to drive. He also struggles with fatigue, which is common with a person with a brain injury. He has some cognitive dysfunction and memory loss. Greg needs time for his brain to heal.

Social Services became involved with Greg's case when he was a patient at Victoria General. The social worker made arrangements to have a caseworker from Social Services come to meet with me at the hospital. He was to discuss a means to financially assist Greg. The worker (he still handles Greg's case) entered Greg's hospital room to view his condition. At that time, I had to fill out information pertaining to Greg's financial status and provide them with a bank statement. Greg's net worth amounted to two hundred and fifty dollars.

He had recently graduated with a certificate in Human Resource Management along with a marketing diploma. He was working at various jobs until he found something in his field. It was determined that Greg would receive the maximum amount of five hundred and ninety-six dollars a month. This would cover his rent of three hundred and eighty, fifty for student loan, food, clothing, and telephone. The relief I felt was short-lived.

I was contacted at the rehab hospital and informed that the hospital was considered my son's home and they would allow him just eighty dollars for his toiletries. I couldn't tell my son that his home was a hospital and because of this attack he would lose again. I fought back and a compromise was made, Greg would receive three hundred and eighty a month.

Greg also required extensive dental work because the seizure medication causes deterioration of his teeth. His financial assistance worker gave us forms to complete for emergency dental work, which were to be given to his dentist, these forms were incorrect. New forms were filled out, they were the wrong forms again; with frustration, I took care of the payment.

My son was told to go look for work regardless of doctor's orders because he looks fine.

A letter was sent to Social Services from Greg's physiotherapist to request additional funds for appropriate shoes for therapy. Greg was instructed to go to several retail outlets for written estimates on running shoes, which he did (keep in mind how tiring it is for him) only to be told that no one is allowed more than fifty dollars for shoes. The woman who gave this information to Greg over the phone was very abrupt so he asked for her name. Her response to his question was "Do you want me to spell it?"

I was furious. When I spoke to her, she suddenly found a means to allow Greg the extra money; he had to provide a doctors' request. Somehow the letter from his therapist had not been included in his computer file.

Greg's monthly payment of five hundred and ninety six will soon be cut to five hundred dollars a month because of new government legislation. He has to fill out a form requesting that he be deemed needy and if successful he will maintain the ninety-six dollars again. His life is spent filling out endless forms with no assistance from the workers at Social Services. He sent forms away, to apply for Canada Disability, and then he was told to fill out forms for provincial government disability. His hope is that he will qualify for this disability to give him time to heal and be retrained for employment. Another suggestion was made that he lives with his mother.

Please understand, I love my son and would give him a home if that was his wish. He is twenty-four years old and has very little to cling to except what's left of his self-esteem. He not only suffered a beating on November10th, but he has also felt beaten each and every day since his attack. Politicians wave the banner of 'Victims' Rights ' but, once elected, seem to abandon their promises. Why do the weak always suffer more? Perhaps they have no choice.

Greg is thankful for the Vancouver Island Head Injury Society and the assistance they have provided. He has a loving family and friends who are his advocates but we are all very disillusioned with a system that has failed him miserably.

Dianne Quinn: Wife, Mother, Caregiver, Advocate

Valentine's Day 3k walk

February fourteenth is the day of love. To me, it meant just over three months since the day I almost lost the chance to show my love to those around me. With Allison and I becoming more than friends after she returned from holidays back east, I decided to show my love for her.

I had my usual occupational therapy session in the morning and thought I would walk afterwards to the closest mall to get Allison a little gift. This gift would show her not only my love but also appreciation in what she was doing for me. This would be my first true venture on my own to a place that was quite a walking distance away through busy intersections and crowds of people.

My fatigue was my greatest worry as I was very confident in my walking ability. I had gone to Tonja's, my stepsister's, boyfriend's Super Bowl party and had to leave at half time due to the noise of the game and partygoers, the stimulation was too much for me to bear. The mall being a mile and a half plus away and me being exhausted after a two-block walk to and from the rehabilitation hospital raised such a concern.

Allison was off job-hunting for the day and I knew she would not be too keen on my attempted feat even though receiving a Valentine's Day gift, so I kept my plan to myself.

My occupational therapy ended and I started my walk home. I came to the intersection where, if I went straight, I would be home in five minutes or turn right and begin a mile and some walk. I never faced such a decision. I would turn right and not even bat an eyelash but now it was a tough choice.

As I stood at the traffic light, I became irritated because such contemplation came from being assaulted and suffering a brain injury. A leisurely walk to the mall was even in doubt because of some ass or asses had beaten me within an inch of my life. I suffered from Post-Traumatic Stress Disorder (PTSD) as anxiety was created by decisions that I linked to my traumatic event. PTSD played its part in my recurring anger.

"Ah, what the heck!" I muttered to myself, turning and going right.

I was on my way. This was going to be a great test for my stamina and endurance.

I was about ten minutes into my walk when I heard the cries of a crow.

When I first moved out west, my second day to be exact, I was attacked by a crow. Looking back maybe some sort of a sign. With this reminder, not only did I look behind me every five steps, a habit I developed walking alone outside, but I also looked up to the sky. People driving or walking by must have thought I was crazy but how were they supposed to know why I was acting this way?

I was accepting of their ignorance, not of the government's. At my last meeting with my financial assistance worker, I gave him articles regarding symptoms of brain injury, along with my doctor and therapists' letters from my initial meeting, but to no avail. The worker did not change my status. Therefore my financial assistance remained the same. My struggles with the government did not help my PTSD, as it seemed I had to rehash November tenth for them to realize something was wrong with me.

I came to the last busy intersection before the mall and pressed the walk across button. I looked to the left and noticed the white walking man sign was lit, so I took a step forward. Before my foot hit the pavement, a car horn had sounded. I stopped and stepped back onto the sidewalk, realizing I was about to walk in front of traffic, paying attention to the wrong perpendicular pedestrian signal.

"Watch it dick!"

The driver, who used his car horn, was slowed by the sudden hit to his brakes and was able to voice such a statement. I turned and faced the direction I was going and waited for the walk across signal.

After close to two hours of walking, I made it to my destination. I went to the jewelry section of a popular department store, looking at sterling silver rings. For a working person reasonably priced, for me, with my budget, the sacrifice of a couple of meals would be necessary. I would have a bowl of cereal as meal replacements. A ring with two hearts intertwined caught my eye. I thought of my sacrifice and decided being hungry and having Cheerios for lunch and supper was worth it.

I bought the ring and put the ring and its box into a small gift bag I also had purchased. I placed the bag in my right hand because my left was starting to tremble. My whole left side would begin to vibrate when I started to become tired. Due to receiving damage predominantly to the right hemisphere of the brain, my left motor functions were affected. I then thought to myself, I was only half way through my walk. I pressed on, looking at my gift and knowing the work I put into it. Allison's reaction also motivated me to push on.

I made it home successfully, requiring a five-hour nap instead of my usual two to three. I would get used to this walk, as my financial assistance worker's office was located in the office building beside the mall. Why mail forms when you are only a bit of a walk away?

5 Hours: 35 Minutes: 25 Seconds

CHAPTER FOUR

On the Mark

My recovery could be best described as miraculous. I was starting my second month of outpatient therapy and I continued to get stronger, physically and mentally. My fatigue was still an issue and I started to accept that it could be everlasting. I still needed eight to ten hours of sleep, not including a two to three hour nap in the afternoon. I would try and wean myself off sleep but, through my sessions with my other health care professionals, I was told to continue to put rest first.

"Hello, Beth."

"Hello, Greg."

Beth was my outpatient physiotherapist.

"I thought we would try the trampoline today. What I will get you to do is take off your shoes and run on the spot. Step up on the trampoline."

"Sure."

The trampoline was about twice the size of a manhole cover. Beth focused on my balance and endurance the previous month. She would sit me on a therapy ball, a large inflated thick rubber ball, have me close my eyes, and allow me to balance myself. When I first attempted such when I closed my eyes, it gave me the sensation as if I were on a roller coaster. Through repetition, this sensation went away and I moved to standing on a wobble board.

Like its name, the wobble board tested your balance, shifting and transferring your weight to mid line. If not, it worked like a teeter-totter and dropped to the side that carried the greatest weight. Again through repetition, I conquered the wobble board.

Along with such balance activities, Beth had me ride the stationary bike. I began at five minutes duration and was now up to twenty minutes.

"Okay, Greg. Ready?"

"Yep."

I started to run on the trampoline. The action of running felt awkward. My legs seemed much heavier than when I walked. Running meant the instructions I used for when I walked had to be increased. Walking had become a subconscious movement for me. I had to recall those steps and multiply them. I was having difficulty registering this and my running seemed staggered and unbalanced.

"Take your time, Greg," Beth said, seeing I was becoming flustered.

After about two minutes, I was able to create a steady stride and rhythm.

"Good, Greg. Can you look to the left for me?"

I did but stopped running.

"Okay now what?" I asked as I stared to my left.

"Greg, I want you to keep running as you look to the left or whichever side I tell you to look to."

"Ohh, okay."

It dawned on me that I was to do two things at once – run and look either to the left or right. I started to run again with less time needed to get going.

"Look to the right," Beth said.

I stopped again, looking to the right.

"Ah shit! Opps, sorry."

I began to run again.

"Look to the right," Beth instructed.

I wanted to stop but did not. There was a dramatic 'hitch' in my stride, but I continued on while looking to the right. After about three times, the stutter step in my running was gone.

"Okay, Greg, that is good. I shall see you on Thursday."

"Yep."

"Before you leave, I want you to have a sit down and rest."

"Yes, I am going to as I am having coffee with Bob."

Beth knew of Bob as he had met me outside the gym earlier and I told her of him.

"Okay. Take care."

"You as well."

I learned in occupational therapy about multitasking and divided attention and saw a problem with these during my run and look to one side trampoline activity. But I also knew these problems would lessen and, with my ongoing progress in my recovery, I began to develop greater self-esteem.

My coffees with Bob also played a large part in this. Bob and I would converse for hours and he would tell me to assist others who had trouble with drinking a beverage or consuming a snack in the cafeteria where we met. Helping others like this was new to me and it felt amazing.

Whenever I finished a therapy session, I was excited to go to Bob. It became innate to walk to the cafeteria and look to the right for him.

Strides

I walked into the hospital for physiotherapy, my first with my new shoes. I was happy about them but also sad knowing someone else had to fight for me to get them. I was looking forward to connecting with Erin, an advocate from the head injury society, in the hope that she would help me fight some of my battles on my own.

"Good afternoon, Beth."

"Good afternoon, Greg. Nice shoes."

"Thanks."

"How are you feeling? Any aches, pains or dizziness since our last session?"

"No. I feel fine."

"The reason for my concern is I had troubles sleeping since the last time we met. I can't believe I had you running. I have not seen someone recover as you are, especially taking into account your trauma. It is very miraculous. Therefore, today, I thought we would concentrate on higher level balance activities so I know when you are running you are safe."

"Sure."

Beth took a sturdy wooden bench, which was about six feet in length, and turned it on its side. Once on its side, Beth made me step up on to it. It was like a balance beam with a width of four inches.

"Okay, Greg. I want you to walk to the end of it."

"Okay."

I began, putting my hands out like I was on a tightrope, even though a foot off the ground. One of my feet fell off a couple times but, in the end, I steadied myself. When I turned and began the balance act back, I had no falls. After completing this task once more, Beth took me to the hallway that led to the cafeteria.

"Next I would like you to run to the end of the hallway, turn, and come back. Run into the turn and do not stop till you are in front of me."

"No problem."

"Ready, go."

I ran to the end, slowed my pace to turn and sprinted back. This was the first time I ran freely since my assault or without being on a trampoline with stand by supervision.

"Okay, Greg; one more time."

"Okay."

I completed another 'lap' and stopped in front of Beth. She nodded with approval and amazement.

"That was very good, Greg. I want you to take a five-minute break to rest and then we will go to the stairwell. I am going to have you walk and increase to a run on them."

As I sat, I thought of Beth's session so far. We started with a difficult balance activity, then I ran, and now I was going to run the stairs. The stairs was a combination of the two activities we had just completed. I became more aware of what my therapy was doing for me and what it tested. I found this very fascinating.

After running up and down two flights of stairs, twice, my session with Beth was finished.

"See you next week, Greg."

"Thanks, Beth. You have a good weekend."

After my coffee with Bob, I exited the hospital. After two steps, I stopped, touching my toes and did a couple of squats. Once upright after my last squat, I began to run.

Seeds

John, my social worker, was able to get the funding for me to see a psychologist for six sessions. John felt I had underlying issues affecting me and that I should speak to a professional who dealt with them. Going to a 'shrink' did not bother me. My mother had gone to one when things were difficult with my father and it made her stronger and allowed her to cope.

My mother and I drove up to the 'Loss Clinic', which appeared to be a large two-story home with a parking lot as its side yard. The waiting area consisted of a few chairs and a stack of outdated magazines located on a small coffee table. The perception of sitting on a leather couch and being asked extremely personal questions lifted as soon as Robin entered the room. Mom, being there as always, made things comfortable from the start.

Something happening to mom, Allison or any family member was stuck in my mind. I had the thought of the benefit of passing away on the bridge I was found on by that passer-by, not having to experience what they did with me. This is selfish of me but I hoped Robin could help me with my mortality issue.

Robin greeted mom and me, with two small dogs following close behind. She introduced them, Pepper, a small shaggy white one, and Toby, a black one of similar traits.

"Okay, Greg, come with me."

I got up and followed as mom reached for one of the magazines. My session was one hour long and mom would wait, something she did not mind doing, knowing I was getting help. As I shut the door, I said to myself, 'Shit something better not happen to her.'

"Well, Greg, get comfortable. That couch has a recline function and a foot rest will spring up by using the lever on the side."

"Thanks."

I pulled the lever up and was comfortable. The lighting in the room was dim but cozy as the blinds were closed and the lamp gave off a warm, inviting feel. I also was surprised that Robin did not have a pen and a notepad.

"Okay, Greg, what can you tell me about what happened to you?"

"Well, this could be a problem. I do not remember anything. I can tell of what happened to me from what I have heard."

One of the small dogs, Toby, seemed to sense my uneasiness as he jumped up onto my lap, lying there for me to caress him. I would later find out Toby went to school for such behavior as he was a certified therapy dog.

"What have you heard?"

"I know I was walking home from my cleaner's job on November tenth, around four thirty in the morning. During this walk, I was assaulted, receiving a brain injury from all the blows to my head. I spent fifteen days in a coma and went through extensive rehabilitation and continue with out-patient therapy today."

"Is there anything that bothers you of this retelling?"

"Well, I did find out I was found on the other side of the street, one I am not usually on. And," I had to take a deep breath as my emotions were taking control from what I was about to say, "I wonder why they did not throw me from that bridge? Right now I have this feeling that I wish they did because I do not ever want to go through such with my mother or a loved one."

"Firstly, Greg, it can be assumed you saw something that made you cross to the other side of the street. Secondly, your perpetrators probably saw a car or something that made them run off. The account you told and the answers to your questions are what you can believe happened and can stick to unless proven otherwise. As for your feelings of mortality, it is part of the grieving process. Do you believe in something beyond here?"

"God-wise?"

"Yes, a higher power."

"I do but really do not know, especially now with what has happened to me."

"I am going to give you a book to read. It is based on Christian philosophies that look into one's mortality. I am not trying to sway you towards a certain belief; I will rather give you a view or insight that may help you."

"Thanks."

"Is there anything else that concerns you?"

"Well, I am extremely exhausted."

"Having suffered a traumatic brain injury, Greg, the energy supply you previously had has been used up to recover. All of us have an energy reservoir that is about the size of a basketball. Yours has been reduced to the size of a grapefruit. For this reservoir to be restored, you must rest and focus on resting. Exerting what little energy you have on thinking of who, what, where, how and why of your trauma will diminish your chances of restoration and result in greater fatigue. Greg, the sad thing is you may not gain back the energy reservoir you once had before your assault. By talking with me and dealing with the trauma, we can try to get by it and put our focus and energy on positive things."

I had lot of information to digest but I understood. The session with Robin was very helpful. Putting a story to November tenth and trying not to focus on the horrific event itself was the greatest help to the initial session. Desensitizing, accepting, and adapting my life to what November tenth brought me would be energy well spent. I hoped I had enough to do so.

CHAPTER FIVE

Expanding

It was the end of another successful month of therapy. I was meeting with John, my social worker, to discuss how I was doing. I felt I had the ability to do more with my spare time. My fatigue was still very prevalent but I was starting to adapt and live with it. I wanted to go beyond the hospital and test myself in the busy world.

I also knew I had a lot of issues with the government and felt like I could handle it on my own. I knew I could not but did not want to put the burden on my mother whenever an issue would arise. These two items were going to be my focus with John.

"Good day, Greg."

"Hello, John."

"How are things going?"

"With therapy, great."

"I have heard from your therapists things are moving along rather nicely."

It was nice to know the therapists felt this way as well and that my recovery was continuing. Being a perfectionist, it was great to have the positive reinforcement.

"How are things outside these walls?"

"I am glad you asked. My difficulty with the government continues and I feel if I knew how to approach them, it would be less of a hassle."

"Is there anything else? How do you spend your time at home? I know you need your down time, but how is your fatigue?"

"I still need my nap in the afternoon but then I am good till bed, which is at about nine o'clock."

"Would you be interested in doing volunteer work? This would be a great way to gauge how you react to a fuller schedule in your day."

"Sure."

"I know of this retirement home that would like someone to call bingo on Tuesday nights. It runs from seven to eight thirty at night. There is no pressure. If you feel uncomfortable after the first time that is fine."

"I will give it a try."

"Also, I would like to introduce you to Erin who I mentioned to you before. She is an advocate with the Vancouver Island Head Injury Society. In fact, they have a support group here at the hospital once a month, and their get-together for this month holds in five days' time. If you would like to attend, I will notify her and she can meet you at the front entrance."

"Sure."

John was very cognizant of brain injury and he knew I struggled with meeting new people and may start to isolate myself. These two options were less intimidating in that one was with people who had my disability in common; the other was with the elderly, a less threatening population.

"I will talk to the retirement home, Brunswick House, and by the end of this week, you can come to my office after therapy or when you visit Bob, and get the specific details."

John was familiar with Bob as he had known of our relationship from when I was admitted and that our friendship was ever growing. I would later find out Bob would use John to check in on me. Even though Bob was not a family member and John could not reveal any personal information, he would tell him of my improvement.

"The next time I see you will be to pick up information and at that time we will set up another date for us to meet next month."

"How's Friday at ten o'clock?" I suggested.

"Sounds good. See you then."

"See you later."

I wrote this in my day-planner, something Paula my OT suggested I use, back when I was an inpatient. Even though my memory was unaffected, I was obsessed with keeping track of everything. I was very organized, to the point of creating more fatigue. All these new events, the places, the times and dates, overwhelmed me a bit but I was vigilant, I had my day-planner.

Others

Allison was nice enough to come with me to the Vancouver Island Head Injury Society's support group/meeting, even though we were growing apart as boyfriend and girlfriend. John, my social worker, set it up so that Erin, an advocate for the head injured and who was a major part of the society, would meet me inside the hospital front entrance. Still, it was nice of Allison to tag along because I was very uneasy of meeting all these new people, including Erin.

Once we stepped into the hospital front entrance, we were met by a bohemian styled woman, about five years older than us. I found her style of 'less is more' very attractive. We made eye contact.

"Greg?" she questioned.

"Erin?" I responded back.

"Nice to meet you. I am glad you could make it to our support group."

"Glad to be here."

A bit of a fib as I was more uncomfortable than I thought I would be. After introducing Allison, we walked to a conference room which had a large table surrounded by people sitting at it; some in wheelchairs, some with walkers or canes beside them. I was taken aback when we stepped into the room, from the different appearances of the people. I knew we all had head injury in common, but after that the differences were many, from a young lady in a power wheelchair to an older gentleman in a suit. Not just by appearance, as I was about to find out.

Allison and I sat at the table and I nodded a hello to a couple of people. Erin situated herself at the head of the table and began to speak.

"Good evening, everyone. We will start with how we usually begin our meeting, going around the table, introducing who you are and background and any difficulties that may have arisen over the past month."

I was happy we went clockwise around the table with the introductions, which meant I was second to last.

"My name is Melanie. I suffered my head injury from a fall in the shower."

This was all Melanie said, as she seemed more uncomfortable than me. What confused me was how a person who slipped in the tub would be in a wheelchair and quite physically impaired.

"My name is George." Unlike Melanie, George was loud and abrupt in his speaking. "I was riding my bike delivering newspapers when a dog ran under me, causing me to fly over the handle bars and hitting my f--king head."

"George," Erin spoke softly to warn him of his language.

"That is all," George replied.

The stories went on with each person having a 'quirk' in their delivery of them. And the problems each encountered made me look inward at the problems I was having. Stupid and miniscule were the adjectives that best described my problems, as we made our way around the table.

An unsettling anger was beginning to grow inside of me. This anger was different from previously, inward anger at myself. How can I complain about monetary issues or relationship issues with Allison when one of the poor souls at the meeting graphically described how he could not make it to the washroom in time; and it was not to urinate.

Hearing the fate of fellow persons with a brain injury also made me realize how fortunate I was. This added increased pressure for me to succeed because I was given a second chance. Apply this to the pressure of meeting mine, and society's expectations before my injury, and it felt like I had the weight of the world on my shoulders.

"Hi. I am Greg. I suffered my head injury from an assault."

Before we moved on to the next person, Melanie asked me a question.

"Why?"

"I do not know. I remember walking home from work and then waking up from what seemed to be a night's sleep. Turned out I awoke from a fifteen-day coma."

"Did they rob you?" Melanie asked.

"No. The police said it was a random act of violence. Wrong place at the wrong time I guess."

"That sucks," she said emphatically.

I was moved by her concern. It was heartfelt. I was starting to become less uncomfortable. Melanie's small token of support made me feel good. After a discussion led by Erin that took into account the problems brought up, the meeting ended. Coffee, soda, and snacks were brought in and we were allowed to mingle.

Surprisingly, I was not shy with talking to other persons. The more I interacted with them, the more comfortable I became. I also became aware of how blessed I was as others may have suffered less tragic circumstances in receiving their brain injury, but were left with greater disability.

Before I left, Erin took me aside and set up a time for us to meet one to one at the head injury society's office. She wanted me to come in and see where the society's offices were located, what else they provided, and discuss any other issues I may have. I learned a lot from the support group and that first meeting. I would be a regular and would lend my support to other persons with a brain injury. With the recovery I received, it was the least I could do.

Lost and Found

Being a part of a crime gives a person certain rights. I was allowed a copy of the police report, my clothing (evidence that was removed as well as cut from body) and any information regarding the case.

I tried to piece together what happened that early morning from these and from my sessions with my psychologist Robin. Robin had stated, 'Believe what I thought happened unless something is revealed to prove otherwise.' For the police, such a way of handling a case would definitely create a reasonable doubt.

The police and detectives on my case were frustrated as more time went by with no significant leads regarding my assault, four other assaults, and a murder, all with the same motive as mine.

When I received the police report, I was not prepared for it. I read the first line and was disturbed. The first line was, Description: assault CBH, which stood for could be homicide. Due to my spontaneous recovery, I did not think I was that close to death until I had read this abbreviation. This reminded me again of how fortunate and blessed I was.

The report then described the scene of the crime. I was located about a third of the way across the bridge, lying supine. I was awake but incoherent and unresponsive. The toque I was wearing was found three feet from my body with one of my gloves close by it. Also found near my hat and glove was a two-inch splinter of wood with my blood on it. The police had the 'K-9' unit, dogs, try and locate the weapon in the brush and trail beneath the bridge but to no avail.

With my attempt at detective work, I made the assumption I was hit by a wood bat or object that knocked my hat off and explained the splinter close by. I could not explain my one glove.

I continued to read and analyze the report. At the end of the bridge where I was found was the entrance to two large apartments/condo complexes, one on each side of the street. These two buildings were run down and had a 'project' feel to them. Both had rowdy parties that evening as the police canvassed the area for witnesses, with some tenants telling of loud music and fights in the hallway. To me, this suggested that I ran into some of the partygoers as they were leaving and they may have become inebriated.

From my clothing, I could not get any clues. My denim jacket had a large bloodstain, determined to be my own, about the size of a pie plate located between my shoulders. This also was a mystery to me as no blood was found elsewhere. Being on the back of the jacket made the stain seem out of place. My clothing also reiterated a mother's advice of wearing clean underwear because the briefs I wore were thread bear and transparent from age and use, with one slight tug of the waist band needed to break them.

The report also described the confusion in my identification. I was amazed by Allison's exact description of my clothing which was the greatest factor in identifying me. I do not think I could recall what a person was wearing an hour after they left brain injury or not.

The last time I spoke to the detectives, they mentioned hypnotherapy (hypnosis) to me and if I was okay to undertake this. A last resort, as I was the only victim of the like crimes who was cognitive enough to do so as the other victims were not so fortunate. After discussing this with my Doctor and Robin my psychologist and given the green light from them, I was comfortable with the idea.

I also wanted to see if any of my analysis of the evidence was true. Closure was not really an issue for me even though I was curious as to what had happened to me. I wanted to prevent this from happening to anyone else.

"Hey, Greg. Snag a seat at my desk," Detective Chabot said.

I had met him and his partner Detective Gannon several times earlier, from the first month in the hospital, which I could not remember, to more questioning, as I recovered.

I sat at the detective's desk, which looked as if a tornado hit it, with files and papers thrown about it. I took notice of three Polaroid pictures clumped together and on top of one of the piles. The three were 'head shots' of a person who looked like they were pummeled by a heavyweight boxer. Upon a closer look, it was I, as a lump formed in my throat as I grabbed them to take an even closer look. Just as I grabbed them, the Detective returned.

"Are these me?" I asked.

"Yes. They were taken by me in the ambulance when you were picked up," he answered in a voice unaffected by them.

Just having them on his desk and in clear view of me made me question his victim impact training.

"Is it okay if I have them?"

"For now."

"Thanks."

I took the three photos and stacked them, placing in my pocket out of sight. I wanted to look over them by myself and grieve the loss they had brought me. I was never asked to give the photos back and still have them today. I will continue to believe my retelling of the events and will likely go to my grave not knowing what happened on the early morning hours of November 10, 1996.

CHAPTER SIX

Follower

"Greg, how is your dental work coming along?" Bob asked.

Due to my assault, being immobile and not having the strength to give myself a thorough brushing for two months, my teeth deteriorated. My anti-seizure medication also added to this as it caused gingivitis. Upon checkup, it was determined I needed close to seventeen hundred dollars of dental work done. The majority of the cost was caused by the need for a root canal to a molar, which was severely chipped by one of the blows to my head.

My visits with Bob increased. I would have coffee with him every day after therapy and Friday I would go to the rehabilitation hospital just to see him. He listened to me and allowed me to show anger and sadness. He gave me his opinion after I would tell him the situations I encountered. He said he would give me understanding but not sympathy. A point I understood from where he is coming from, literally.

Bob knew of my dental expense as I told of my plight with social services (financial assistance worker/government). I told him at a previous coffee how I had walked up there to get forms for such assistance and had to do it twice as my worker gave me the wrong forms. Bob knew how this tired me. I never used the bus due to all the strangers and not being comfortable around a crowd I did not know. Isolation is a symptom of brain injury.

Turned out all they could provide me with was two hundred and fifty dollars of coverage because it was considered not an emergency. If my teeth were like this during my stay in the hospital, it would have been deemed an emergency and I would have been covered. The government ignored the fact that because of my emergency my teeth were in the shape they were in. Bob had asked me about my teeth earlier, focusing on the cost.

"Well, Bob, mom is going to give me five hundred like I mentioned earlier and, with the two fifty from Social Services, I am going to get seven fifty done. This will cover the work I need at the moment and I will get the rest done when I can afford it. I hope my teeth don't fall out in the meantime."

Upon saying this, Bob slid an envelope across the table.

"What is this?" I questioned.

"A card of thanks, for you coming in to see me."

I opened the envelope to a card, which read thank you for being a friend. I opened the card and there in the sleeve of the card were five one hundred dollar bills. I began to well up with tears and slid the card back across the table to him.

"I can't accept this, Bob."

He then angrily stated as he slid the card back to me, "Take it. I do not want to argue about it. I enjoy giving and sharing. For my enjoyment, you must accept and it will make my day."

"Thank you, Bob. I do not know what to say."

Bob knew I did not have to say a thing but take what he did and learn from it and do the same.

"Well, buddy, it is close to noon, and I have to go back to my room and help feed one of my roommate's lunch. I am starting to enjoy living here because I like helping."

"I know you do," I said, still moved by what he did and has done for me.

As we left the cafeteria and exchanged good byes and when we would meet again, I watched Bob push the wheels of his chair with great force down the hall. He was in a hurry to get back and feed his friend.

He was adapting to his situation better than I was, and helping was a key in his adaptation. This did not surprise me because Bob gives more than those who can walk and are a quarter his age. I know in time I will give it a try and do the same, I was learning.

BOB'S WORDS

Nobody knows what tomorrow brings
By living & giving
And sharing & caring today
Lets one know
That if tomorrow does not come
Today is a good day
To be the last

Angel

I met Sharon through Bob. Like Bob, she lived in extended care. Bob took her under his wing like he did with me and they became close friends. Bob even donated an expensive piece of rehabilitation equipment to the hospital for Sharon to use and in turn for everyone to use.

Sharon was in extended care because she suffered from multiple sclerosis, a horrible, progressive, and disabling disease. The illness took everything away from her but not her loving spirit. She lost the use of arms and legs and was in a power wheelchair controlled by her puffing into a mouthpiece.

I was amazed at Sharon in that she always had a smile on her face and was content with her life and what she was dealt. It did not bother her that someone had to scratch her nose if it itched. She was not bothered with sipping her coffee through a long straw, possibly burning the tip of her tongue. She just loved being with Bob and me, listening and conversing.

"So Greg, you seem down," Sharon said, as it was just the two of us, as Bob had to leave for his acupuncture.

"Ahh, Sharon, I am just pissed off with the ignorance people have towards me and I am sure others with mental, invisible disabilities."

My trials with my financial assistance worker (FAW) and the government, most recently getting quotes for the new running shoes I wore, were increasing and getting worse. I had a feeling that my FAW continued to judge me on my physical appearance disregarding what I went through and was going through, thinking I should be over it by now. He was not in my shoes, pun intended.

"Greg, can I tell you a story?"

"Definitely."

I always was an eager listener to what Sharon or Bob had to say to me. Like Bob, I was in awe with how she handled her situation. If I were in her situation, I do not think I could carry on let alone handle it the way Sharon did.

"I remember when I was first diagnosed with multiple sclerosis. I progressively got worse, losing the use of one leg, then both legs, and then my arms. Of course at first I did not want to accept it. I struggled with walking and did not want to even use a cane. I remember being in the grocery store and stumbling, falling into things. I looked back and there were these ladies who were amused by me, thinking I was intoxicated. As they walked by, I informed them why I stumbled and what caused it. I was not proud of being short with them, but they were ignorant of my disease. Greg, it hurts accepting that you have a problem but telling people so they do not judge you without knowing what is wrong takes their power of ignorance away."

"Thank you, Sharon."

"You are welcome. It will be tougher Greg, for people to see and accept your illness. Physically, you are fine. When I started using a cane, then walker, and then wheelchair, the ignorance decreased and stopped."

What an amazing person saying that it would be tougher for me, being the way she is. I would visit Sharon as much as Bob as the two seemed inseparable. In fact, there was a rumor that the two were an item, which was impossible as they were both happily married. I had met their two wonderful, caring spouses during my many visits.

Rumors and gossip spread in extended care like anywhere else. I guess with rumors and gossip it felt like the outside world, away from a place where they would spend the remainder of their lives.

I loved going to the Gorge for not only rehabilitation but also for my coffees. I not only improved with my therapy but also improved spiritually, because of my two best friends. A wheelchair-bound seventy-eight-year-old man and middle-aged woman with a disabling disease. Who would have thought that my closest friends would hold such traits? God did.

Favorite Game

Brunswick House could be best described as a retirement home for the elite. Seeing how Bob and other elderly lived in extended care, in comparison to this, was like a soup kitchen compared to a five-star hotel. I just wished there was a system in place that allowed all the aged to live comfortably and not have such extremes.

I was dressed in khakis, a golf shirt, and dress shoes. I viewed this first day of volunteering as that of a new job. John, my social worker, coordinated this as he knew the importance of me not isolating myself as persons with a brain injury have a tendency to do.

I was met at the front door of this lavish, four-story building by Dani, the coordinator of activities at Brunswick. He would show me around the residence and tell me the rules of calling Bingo. He showed me where the bingo cards and turn-able bin with balls, which had numbers and letters on them, were located.

Once we grabbed the necessary bingo equipment, we went into a large room, which had five tables each surrounded by four chairs. At the front of the room was a smaller table with chair. This was for the bingo caller, me.

After setting up my area, Dani told me the rules. Each bingo card cost one quarter, with a player allowed to purchase a maximum of four cards. We would play four rounds. A one line, a two line, the letter 'X', and a full card; with each subsequent game given a greater prize amount, with the full card receiving the greatest jackpot. I was familiar with bingo 'lingo' as my older sister Kim and I use to play every once in a while in Windsor when I lived there.

Once Dani went over the rules, the residents began to trickle in. The residents I made eye contact with greeted me with a warm smile, some mouthing the word 'hello'. After about five minutes, the room was full and Dani spoke.

"Good evening, everyone. We have a new caller. His name is Greg and he has volunteered to call our bingo for the next little while. So, let's welcome him and assist him as he gets used to us and bingo."

I heard several hellos when Dani stopped his introduction. He then helped me give out cards and collect the money for them.

"Okay, Greg. You all right? I am stepping out."

"Yep."

I was okay, but anxiety ran through my body. It felt like I was doing a business presentation at college, only multiplied by ten.

"Good evening, folks. As Dani stated, I am Greg and I will be your caller for this evening," my voice shaking from nerves.

One of the residents, Trudy, looked at me and winked, quietly telling me not to be nervous.

"The first game we will be playing is for one line. It can be horizontal, vertical, or diagonal. The winner will receive one dollar and fifty cents."

The first two games dragged a bit but, by the third, I was calming down and enjoying my new job. After bingo was shouted, we started the last game of the evening, a full card for five dollars. A jackpot of five dollars drew some 'ohhhs' from the crowd.

"Our next letter and number is B six."

"What is the letter?" a cute little lady asked from the table in front of me.

"B," I answered.

"The letter?"

I was a bit dumbfounded and stated B again. The lady then turned to her friend beside her and asked, "Why won't he tell me the letter?"

Her friend then replied with "six" and she responded with "Thank you," glaring at me with a look I thought could not be produced by someone so cute.

Whoa I thought to myself, I was a bit amused, however. I continued on with the game and overheard the little lady tell her friend she did not like the new caller.

"O 64."

"Bingo."

Sure enough it was the player who was not impressed by my calling skills. As I gave her the five dollars for the bingo, she said, "You are the best caller."

"Thank you," I replied.

After cleaning up and mingling with the residents, I started my bus ride home. I had to transfer and switch buses downtown. I was not nervous about my bus ride home and being downtown after dark. I was lost in thought of my first evening calling bingo and the sometime strange comical interactions I experienced. I was taken away from the fears brought on by my ordeal and concentrated on something positive, helping others. It made me want to do more.

CHAPTER SEVEN

Spotting Me

I was excelling at my therapies and the talk of discharge from out-patient therapy was being discussed amongst my health care team. My physiotherapist, Beth, made the suggestion of getting a membership at a fitness center. She was aware of my weight training and active lifestyle prior to my incident and felt I was at a stage in my recovery to reintroduce this back into my life, albeit slowly.

My occupational therapist Edith also liked this suggestion as she noticed I was improving socially and going out to a different environment was a way to continue with my growth outside the hospital. Bingo and the support group were increasing my confidence and comfort around others.

I went to the Community Recreational Center, located about a thirty minutes' walk away from my apartment, for my first attempt at lifting weights again. Like everything else, I had to go through a bureaucracy of filling out forms and a letter stating my need for financial assistance.

Surprisingly, the results of such cumbersome, redundant actions were to my benefit as I received a three-month membership free of charge. The receptionist was thoughtful and showed concern towards my ordeal and said she would grant me another three months if I needed it.

This was a first in the many people I had dealt with, with regard to assistance financially. It was because Rhona, the recreation center administrator who I dealt with, had compassion, something the workers of the government seemed to be lacking.

I went into the weight room, really not knowing how my body would react to lifting weights. I knew not to be upset or disappointed by what I could do because I was half the person I was muscularity wise compared to the person before my ordeal. I also knew my stamina needed work as my fatigue continued to be an ongoing problem, as medium distance walks to the grocery store required me taking a nap afterwards.

Whenever I did work out at a gym, I adhered to the proper weight room etiquette. I would put weights back after use, wipe machines down after I had used them, and let others work in with me if they wanted to.

The gym that day was empty other than a young lady and a muscular built older man. I made sure I let him use the machines before me because, now more than ever, I wanted to avoid any confrontation. And by the looks of this fellow, I definitely did not want to piss him off by holding him up or him tripping on a weight I left unattended.

I set up the curl bar with about a third of the weight I used to be able to lift. After putting on the weight, I let the big guy go by.

"Excuse me," I said as I took two steps forward to let him by.

He said nothing and sat on the padded bench located beside me and continued on with his workout. I mouthed the word "Okay" to myself and bent over to pick up the curl bar.

As I lifted the weight and started to curl, my right arm had no problem with curling the bar, but my left side struggled with the curl so much so I teetered over to get the bar caught up and even with my right side. I did not stop and kept at it. I knew this would happen because the most severe blow was to the right side of my head leaving my left side affected and weaker. It frustrated me, but the only way to improve was from repetition, something I learned from therapy. After five repetitions, I set the bar down and sat at the bench behind me. I looked in the mirror, which covered the entire wall in front of me, and noticed the built man looking at me. I smiled at him and, before I started another set, he spoke.

"Are you all right? I noticed you struggled with that last rep."

"Yes, thanks. It is from a brain injury but in time it will improve."

"I hope it does. I will pray for you."

Before I could respond with a thank you, I was startled by the fact that this intimidating stranger would say such a thing. After a short pause, I thanked him for such a wonderful statement and introduced myself.

"By the way, my name is Greg."

I put out my hand to shake his and he put out his to shake mine.

"My name is Phil. If you don't mind me asking, how did you receive your head injury?"

"No, I don't mind. I was walking home from work and someone attacked and struck me from behind."

Robin's therapy, which focused on desensitizing me to what happened, along with the support group, paid dividends as I did not get upset telling of my incident to Phil. My psychologist's last session was a couple weeks ago, and her idea of me establishing a relationship with a church was put on the back burner as I was not impressed about going to a place filled with complete strangers, but now I had an opening and, with my new ever growing confidence amongst strangers, was less afraid.

After Phil had commented on how horrible my incident was, I asked him about his statement earlier.

"You said you would pray for me?"

"Yep, I will. I have been through some tough times myself, and God helps."

"I could not agree with you more," I said.

I then explained to Phil about how I was new to the area and had not established a relationship with a church yet, and wondered if he had any suggestions.

"Well, Greg, if you want, you can meet me and my family at our church. It is a Baptist church called Lambrick Park."

After giving me directions, I said good-bye to Phil and that I would see him on Sunday. The thought of going to a place filled with strangers did not bother me anymore. Phil was a stranger.

Interdependence

I went into the church and was met by Phil at the front door. The building did not have the traditional structure associated with a church and looked more like a convention center.

"How are you, Greg?"

"Good, thanks."

Phil then handed me a plastic bag and within it was a homemade loaf of bread.

"Thank you."

"You are welcome."

Phil did not know of my struggles with the government and that sometimes good food at times was hard to come by for me. Being a young man, I had my pride and did not want to rely on others. This drove my mother nuts as she wanted to help and I was becoming more willing to accept her help as I knew struggling unnecessarily was not to my benefit.

"This is a big place," I said to Phil.

"It's a big congregation of about 500," Phil replied.

There were no pews but rows of chairs that were linked together. There were three sections, left, center, and right. Phil, his wife, and two kids were in the right section close to the front of the stage. I noticed the left section near the back had an empty row and told Phil I would like to sit there by myself. He was not offended and said to meet him after the service as he wanted to have me over for lunch and give me a drive home.

The service began with wonderful worship music. The music was not carried out by a solo singer at an organ but a whole band composed with a guitarist, drummer, and several vocalists. The hymns as well as newer Christian based songs were projected on to a big screen at the front of the auditorium. The congregation all stood as we all sang together.

I never experienced such worship music as I was brought up in the Lutheran church and the hymns were sung in unison from a very old hymnal book located at the bottom back of the pew in front of you.

The music washed over me and I felt like I was not alone. In the literal sense, I was not, as a young man, close to my age, sat near me. After a few songs, we sat down again, with the young man a couple empty seats to my right-hand side. We glanced at each other, giving the obligatory head nods hello.

The sermon was about giving and accepting gifts and learning to do the same. I was astonished at how the sermon hit home, it felt like it was meant for me to hear. The sermon lasted for about thirty minutes and the service ended with two more songs by the worship team.

I stood with the stranger located two seats down from me, when on the last song the lead vocalist told the congregation to join hands. I looked to my left and then my right and it was just me and the stranger in the row, making this request seem very awkward. We looked at each other, and each of us nodded a look of what the heck while shrugging our shoulders. We side-stepped and held hands.

After the song and final prayer, the service ended. Before meeting up with Phil, I introduced myself to the stranger who I had an unexpected duet with.

"That was interesting. I am Greg," I said, offering my hands out to shake his.

"I am Sam," he said while chuckling.

We exchanged phone numbers and, in the months to come, Sam and I became close friends. He would treat me to dinners and give me a place to stay when things were not going well with Allison. I would meet another great friend through Sam, his best friend Brian, and years later would attend Sam's wedding in Edmonton, Alberta.

God introduced me to Phil, then Sam and Brian. And these strangers as well as others would provide me support that allowed me to become independent again.

My turn

Erin from the head injury society was able to connect me with a person who coordinated services for people with special needs. Erin mentioned an opportunity to help another person with a brain injury with an aquatics class. I would meet up with him once a week for the next six months and assist him with an exercise program/class that took place in the pool.

My initial meeting with Vincent startled me, to put it mildly. I met him at the recreation center that housed the pool and expected someone similar to me. He was not as he was using a walker to help with his walking and he had speech difficulties, with me having to ask him to repeat what he had said many times to understand him when we conversed.

This showed me the varying outcomes of traumatic brain injury. I was somewhat aware of them from attending the support group at the Gorge and recently at a survivor barbeque set up by the society when one individual in attendance urinated in front of us thinking he was in the bathroom.

After our first and initial class, I was able to support Vincent with the class successfully. I was surprised at the support I had to provide him from assisting with undressing and getting ready for the class to getting into the pool helping him with certain exercises to then showering and getting dressed afterwards.

Looking back, I thought how risky it was for me and Vincent to have done the classes as I was only six months post my injury and my balance was okay but having to assist someone on slippery surfaces with their walking and entering and exiting a pool would not have been something Tracey, Lou, and Beth, my physiotherapists, would have suggested.

This volunteering also showed me how services for those with a brain injury may be lacking as Vincent was reliant on me, a fellow person with a brain injury, to support him.

Over the several classes we did over the few months, I developed a friendship with Vincent as in our second to the last time together we discussed and decided to go out for lunch after our following week's last aquatics class. My mom and Brian, my step father, wanted to meet Vincent and treat both of us to a nice meal.

I decided to move in with mom and Brian in Powell River, British Columbia in a couple months and needed time to tie up loose ends, moving and dealing with the bureaucracy of the government and the support they provided me. I gave the coordinator who organized our time together a month's notice as I wanted Vincent to find someone else to support him.

It was 9:15 when I arrived at the recreational center, my usual time of arrival which gave us forty-five minutes to get change and ready for the class. When I arrived with my tote bag in hand which contained my swimwear and towel, I was surprised to see Vincent very well dressed and with no tote bag.

I was about to question where his change of clothes were but did not, I realized he forgot that we would swim first and then go out for lunch. Vincent was always punctual for our classes together and was again this week, but adding the event of going out for lunch afterwards was too much for him to remember, making him forget that we had aquatics first.

I called mom from a payphone and she and Brian would do their best to see if they could arrive earlier.

"Hey, Vincent."

"Hey, Greg."

"Just got off the phone with my mom and step dad. They are running late, so we have over an hour or so to kill. Would you like a coffee?" As I placed my tote bag out of sight under the table.

"Sure."

I purchased coffee for us, and we sat, not saying much.

I heard the honk of Brian's car and Vincent and I made our way to the car. Mom had a look of sadness and pride as I assisted Vincent into the backseat and did his seat belt up. As we drove to the restaurant, mom and Brian conversed with Vincent and were able to understand him even though they had to repeat to verify what he said a few times as I told them of his communication issues.

We made our way into the restaurant and to our seats with me situating myself close enough to assist Vincent if he needed help. When our food arrived, I cut Vincent's food into smaller pieces. We would have lunch a few times at the cafeteria after swim class and I noticed the struggles he sometimes had with swallowing.

The meal was great, and not much was said.

"How is your food? " I asked.

"Great, this is heaven," Vincent responded.

I looked around the table and mom, Brian, and I were becoming teary-eyed. This man who struggled to walk five feet and required great assistance to take a basic aquatics class pointed out how a simple meal in a restaurant was heavenly. The perspective gained from this was not lost on me or mom and Brian.

The dinner went by quickly and we drove Vincent to his apartment. When we arrived, I took him up, with mom and Brian waiting in the car for me to return.

He unlocked his apartment and, when I walked in, was saddened. His apartment was quite cluttered and disorganized. I could have easily been Vincent, and would fight to live on my own as well, even though in his condition it would involve taking great risk, falls being the greatest.

I was overcome with emotion and said good bye and thanked Vincent for our time together. He responded, thanking me, and handed me a clementine from his fridge for the road and I placed it in my coat pocket.

I opened the back door to Brian's car, sitting and doing up my seat belt. Mom and Brian did not say anything as I began to weep, placing my hand into my pocket to hold the small token of appreciation given to me. I now knew I had to do more for others with a brain injury.

CHAPTER EIGHT

Unique

I usually received my government assistance check the last Wednesday of the month. The monetary amount was not enough to get by, but mom would help me. I put my pride aside which being a twenty-four-year-old male was very difficult for me to do.

My mother left two weeks after I was discharged as an inpatient and I had finished my first week of outpatient therapy. She was reluctant leaving, being the amazing and nurturing mother she is but she knew she had to ease up and let me try living on my own with Allison to become independent.

Mom decided to come for a visit three weeks after she had left to see how I was doing. She entered my apartment and was a bit surprised that I looked the same regarding my weight and that I did not gain any weight. She showed me pasta dishes and recipes I could make and handle on my own and reiterated that snacks would be okay at the moment. Some bad snacks included, chocolate bars and chips.

"How are you doing, Greg?"

"Good."

Mom gave my bedroom and the apartment a quick walk through and was happy to see it was clean and in order. She then went to the kitchen.

"Everything is good, mom."

I was trying to distract her from going to the refrigerator but to no avail. When she opened the door and saw the sparse contents, she was not happy and in fact angered. Allison did not eat much, being a petite girl and would usually grab something to eat on the go when running her errands.

"What is this?" she asked, exasperated.

"What? Milk, OJ and liver is in there..." I was trying to give the impression I was getting by.

The three weeks that mom was not there, I was hungry but knew to ration and eat cereal a couple meals a day and would buy liver which was cheap. I did not realize this was not smart, especially for my injured brain which needed nutrients from fruits and vegetables. My brain and body required greater calories more than ever during the early months of recovery and reconditioning.

"Got a question for you, Greg."

"What?"

"So, starving yourself proves what?"

I did not respond.

"Just as I thought, son, I want to help you and know you would help me and pay me back. By not letting me be a mom, you are hurting yourself and me."

What she said hit home. I was very fortunate in the insight I would gain through certain events in my rehabilitation and recovery from brain injury. I remember trying to get from my bed to my wheelchair on my own when I was told by my physiotherapist and health care team that I still needed assistance. When I fell and thankfully was able to get my arms in front of me, preventing another brain injury, I realized I had to wait and follow what I was told. Sadly, with brain injury, some do not gain insights from the consequences of their actions and will continue to try things on their own, not realizing the damage they could cause to themselves. Poor memory also played its part; with me, this did not. I learned my lesson and now was learning another.

I would rely on my mother and the system for support after brain injury. My mother went to the extreme with her help and my financial assistance worker (FAW) did the opposite. And dealing with my FAW was testing me and my anger.

I would see an anger counselor, something my social worker John coordinated. I would see him several times, my sessions being once a week. My anger was not only focused on how I was treated by the government but an inward anger caused by seeing other persons with a brain injury through my support group, volunteering with Vincent and other outpatients I would see in rehabilitation. I was questioning how I came out of my brain injury so blessed and they did not.

The sessions helped as my counselor said I had the right to get angry at things that would usually make anyone angry, and not get angry at myself for getting angry. I thought back to when I was an inpatient in rehab and my mom saying "Greg, look at the other patients" and that I should be grateful. I responded with, "Other people's suffering does not make me feel good."

My anger counselor allowed me to be angry and assisted me with lessening the guilt I felt with getting better in comparison to others. He and John knew I needed to get this inward anger out, from writing and talking to someone.

I started writing in a journal early on in my recovery and through my sessions with Robin my psychologist and now my anger counselor was expressing it vocally. I was now about to become more vocal with the system that did not help me, but minimized the support I needed in the most important year of my life.

Condiment

After nine months of battling my financial assistance worker, I finally lost my cool in a phone call. The 'levy broke' when I found out through Erin, my advocate from the head injury society, of the disability support provided by the provincial government. I was unaware of this and only told of two sections of support given by the government.

I am not proud of the conversation I had with my worker, but the struggles I endured due to him blatantly ignoring my invisible disability in such a crucial first year in recovery from brain injury, even with the loads of information he was given, he had it coming and this angry rant was long overdue. If he would have been transparent and given me the support of someone who was disabled I would have put less of a burden on my mother and the financial support she gave me.

After my heated exchange, more one-sided as my worker stammered to come up with the logic of withholding information, I met with Erin to figure out how I could get this disability designation. We would have to go through a tribunal where we would present my case to a panel of three persons who would come to a decision. The panel would be made up of a government worker, a person with a disability, and an unbiased person.

Erin and I put together a strong case over the month after my fiery call and when we entered the room which had the three panel members, the moderator, and the provincial lawyer, we were confident. My confidence may have been muted by the racing thoughts running through my recovering brain. I still could not believe I was going through this. The date of the tribunal ironically was one week before the one-year anniversary of my assault. The whole year still seemed like a dream, at times more like a nightmare.

Erin spoke eloquently, sharing her vast knowledge on brain injury and the affects brain injury has on a person and their loved ones. She personalized this by using my story and all the advocating she and my mother did for me as an example. As she spoke, I observed the province's lawyer.

He must have been just a few years older than me. I viewed him as what maybe I could have been. I reflected on my educational path and how I failed at university, excelled at college and even with this was frustrated with my choice of business administration as a career.

I never took schooling seriously and viewed those who did as not popular or social. I think back to high school in the 'Soo', out of my small graduating class, four went on to become doctors. The lawyer had to take school seriously and now he was doing great, I am sure. My in the moment self-reflection of what could have been was upsetting me and now I was about to speak.

"Greg," Erin spoke.

I snapped out of my thoughts, "Yep, I just want to begin by thanking you Erin for all that you have done for me and my mother. You helped us through all the bureaucracy and I definitely would not be here today if not for your advocating and help."

I took a deep breath. I really did not plan on saying what I was about to; it just came out, straight from the heart.

"November tenth, the date my life changed. Everything after that date for almost a year now is affected by what happened on that date."

Through my sessions with Robin, my psychologist, I know I suffered from Post-Traumatic Stress Disorder (PTSD) and would research PTSD on my own.

"I was in the grocery store recently. I always loved barbeque sauce, putting it on hamburgers, hot dogs, and dipping my French fries in it. I was in the aisle where they had ketchup, mustard, sauces and spices. I picked up this bottle of mesquite barbeque sauce and thought how tasty it would be. I then looked at the price and had to put it back. I was on a strict, fixed budget."

I began to cry, with Erin placing her hand on my shoulder to comfort me to continue.

"I could not afford eighty cents extra for barbeque sauce because I was nearly beaten to death while walking home from work. This horrific event and what these people did to me was now affecting even the smallest of things, like buying barbeque sauce. I did not ask to be here today or for any of this. I just want my life back and not have to keep on fighting for the simple things. When I do have to fight, I am back fighting those people who assaulted me on November tenth."

I was done speaking and, after some final discussion as to what would happen next, Erin and I left the room. Erin had to get back to her office and the head injury society. The panel would render a decision in thirty minutes so I decided to stay and would contact Erin with the results when I knew. I sat just outside the room and put my head down and began to pray.

"Lord, thank you for allowing me to speak and for all your help. Whatever they decide I accept and I am grateful I had the opportunity to express myself. In your Son's name, amen."

After my short prayer, I looked up and the unbiased panel member gave me an envelope with a smile and stated, "Three to nothing in your favor."

"Thank you so much."

I began to choke up with joy. I would leave the province five months later and, due to not being in British Columbia's jurisdiction, the disability support I should have gotten a year earlier would end. But I was still ecstatic and proud. I set precedent for other persons with a brain injury as they could refer to my case in their fight with the government and receive the financial support they so desperately need, especially early on in recovery from their invisible disability.

For Now

I was leaving Victoria to live with my mother and stepfather Brian in Powell River, approximately five hours away by car and ferry ride. The three of us wanted to have lunch with Bob and say good bye to him and the health care team that was so instrumental in me gaining back my life and begin the process of living independently. I also wanted to say good bye to Sharon.

I was extremely emotionally labile early in my recovery and this is commonplace with brain injury. My brain went from not allowing me to produce emotions early in my recovery displaying a flat affect, to producing emotions at full blast. This would result in laughter at jokes for too long a time, but also weeping to the point of no more tears.

I was preparing for one of these cries with my farewells. I was starting to get a handle on my emotions but for the time being had to tell myself that I had cried or laughed long enough, where before my brain injury this was not required.

After saying good bye to the amazing therapists who gave me my life back, we went to the cafeteria for lunch.

"Hey, Bob."

"Hey, you three. So great to see you."

Bob was sitting in the cafeteria in the extended care portion of the rehab hospital, waiting and holding a table for four. I had many coffees with him and learned so much from our conversations here. Not only did I come after my outpatient therapy which was located right down the hall, but on weekends and other days. He was my best friend and my mentor.

"So, what is the plan?" Bob asked us.

"Going to live with mom and Brian up in Powell River. Stay there till spring and then move back east."

Brian then spoke, "My sister is battling cancer and we would like to be there for her."

"Sorry to hear, Brian. Will pray for you and her."

"Thanks, Bob."

After close to an hour lunch, talking and discussing the memories of the past year, it was time to say good bye. I also wanted to go down the hall to Sharon's room and say good bye.

"Well, Bob, I just want to thank you so much for all that you have done for me."

My mother chimed in, stating how fortunate she was to have Bob keep an eye on me and give me support.

"You are both welcome. I have something for you, Greg."

Before I could respond with 'you have done too much', Bob stood up. My jaw almost hit the floor as Bob stood in front of me. He then took two shuffled and labored steps and we embraced in a hug. This man was given up on and told he would never walk again but through great determination proved the naysayers wrong.

I was trying to keep it together and this was even made more difficult by mom crying and seeing Brian, who is a big man in stature, having large tears roll down his cheeks.

"Love you, Bob."

"Love you too."

After composing myself, I went by myself to see Sharon in her room. Mom and Brian stayed back and continued chatting with Bob and thanking him again for all that he had done for me.

I found Sharon's room and spoke before entering.

"Sharon…"

"Who's there?"

"Greg, just want to say good bye, heading back east."

"Come on in."

Sharon was lying supine in bed and, before approaching her, I looked at the lovely photos on the wall of her room. One was of her family and Sharon was standing in the photo, not in a wheelchair and dealing with the savagery of multiple sclerosis.

"Beautiful picture and family," I stated.

"You know what is missing from the photo, you," Sharon replied.

I did not know how to respond. I walked to the head of Sharon's bed and thanked her for being an amazing friend and for all the advice she gave me. I kissed her on the forehead and told her.

I loved her. She replied with the same.

I walked down the hallway and met up with mom and Brian. As we left the Gorge Hospital, I was grateful I was able to leave. I also was saddened that this could be the last time I saw two of my best friends.

CHAPTER NINE

Applied Knowledge

I was enamored by what the health care professionals did for me in my rehabilitation from a severe traumatic brain injury.

My occupational therapists Paula and Edith who worked on my cognitive deficits caused by brain injury like organization, memory, and sequencing. Paula taught me energy conservation strategies to deal with my fatigue. She also helped and cured my left inattention issues I had suffered from early on in my recovery. Being struck to the right side of my head affected my left side functions and vice versa. This occurs with a majority if not all neurotrauma and with cardio vascular accidents (strokes) as well.

My physiotherapists (PT): Tracey, Lou, and Beth, who stretched my deconditioned legs and got me mobile and not only walking, but running again.

My speech language pathologist (SLP) Marla who taught me how to swallow and made sure I was able to communicate, being able to receive and comprehend information and expressing myself clearly verbally and in writing.

To my social worker John who introduced journaling to me as a way to deal with my anger and from these journals write my story and had this story published years later.

John also prepared me for the outside world and was instrumental in giving me direction after my traumatic brain injury, linking me to Erin and the head injury support group and society. Erin not only gave me support through advocacy but also directed me to do volunteer work with other persons with a brain injury.

And most importantly Bob my beloved friend, the stranger and patient who I first opened up to when I entered rehab. My daily visits with Bob in extended care when I did outpatient rehab taught me and showed me how to care and assist others in need. He led by example and I would follow. When I returned to Ontario in nineteen ninety eight, I would take another year and half off, resting, recovering and volunteering. I would fly out west to visit Bob the next three years and see how he was doing.

I went back to school attending Sault College in my hometown of Sault Ste. Marie, Ontario in the fall of nineteen ninety nine. I attended the

Rehabilitation Assistant Certificate Program which allowed me to assist occupational therapists and physiotherapists. I learned a lot from the fifteen-month program about the health care field and myself.

Going back to school was a true test for me since my assault. I went to the special needs office at the college and explained the concerns I had caused by my brain injury and that fatigue was my greatest issue. The only thing they could do was lengthen the program to two years. I decided against this and to go for it.

The courses and what I learned from them came naturally to me. I applied my own rehabilitation experience to what I was absorbing from my teachers and textbooks. I did discover some limitations caused by my brain injury that saddened me, but knowing them I was able to combat them.

Fatigue was one of the limitations I knew of already. I did an annual neuropsychological test and assessment three times and the results revealed I would have a fatigue problem for the rest of my life. I battled this fatigue as best I could. I slept seven to ten hours a night and took two-hour naps on the weekend.

Before my brain injury and subsequent fatigue, I could go to school full time, have a part-time job, and go out on the weekend and a week night once in a while. Those days were far behind as all the energy I mustered was used to concentrate on my studies, nothing else. In those fifteen months at the college, I gained thirty pounds as I could not go to the gym or go for a jog.

I will not rule out that my fatigue will lessen. I dealt with many specialists in my recovery and rehabilitation from brain injury and remember two differing statements. One being whatever deficits remain after two years would be permanent and ongoing. The other, fifteen years down the road, a function may return or deficit decrease. I am going with the latter even though I am not naïve knowing my fatigue may be permanent.

The two years prior to going back to school, when I gained the ability to do so, I went to the gym, went for a run or a walk. I tried participating in physical activity four times a week. I would not feel the energy at first but would feel more energetic a couple days later, similar to the law of diminishing returns.

Another limitation that revealed itself was my organizational deficit. Organization is an executive function located in the frontal lobe of the brain. I received damage to this lobe as the initial contact and blow to the back of my head caused my brain to move forward and strike the front of my skull, a coup-countrecoup injury in clinical terms. I failed the organization section of the neuropsychological test which annoyed me as I felt I was very organized. I had a day planner, something that my occupational therapist Paula got me hooked on back in rehab and I was always aware of my appointments, giving myself extra time to prepare.

John, my social worker, explained to me that all the steps I took were compensation for my organizational deficit. I needed structure and writing things down, triple checking them, and being prepared gave me this structure. This made sense to me as these steps would become stressful and lead to greater fatigue.

My organizational problem became very evident as the one exam I failed was open book. I did not have a plan, no structure to my studying. Thumbing through the textbook frustrated me to the point that I handed in an empty exam.

Besides dealing with my limitations and gaining the weight, I did enjoy my two years of school and took the spring of two thousand and one off to train for my first marathon. Similar to my education, I focused on running and nothing else. I never thought I could go back to school and run a marathon. Having being stripped of the ability to walk let alone run, and gaining this back influenced my decision to take on such a feat. I was doing things I thought I would never do and knew that positive path my life had taken was created by those who helped me. I now wanted to do the same.

Marathon #1

I took the plastic cup of water from the volunteer's hand. She was cheering me on, yelling 'Awesome you are doing great' along with 'keep it up'. I was coming up to the thirtieth kilometer.

I did not realize the mental struggle involved with running a marathon. The two thousand and one St. John's Ambulance Kitchener-Waterloo marathon consisted of two laps of a twenty-one kilometer course. When I completed lap one, I was exhausted physically and mentally, especially knowing I had to do another lap, and contemplated that I should have done the half marathon.

I trained hard for this day as I took a three-month break after I completed college and thought the best way to get in shape would be to train and complete a marathon as I had gained about thirty pounds during my studies.

I followed a schedule from a running magazine but made a huge error, I mistook kilometers for miles, so instead of three miles a day for training I would do three kilometers. I was now feeling the error of my ways.

I hit kilometer thirty-two and said to myself, "Just ten more."

I did a ten-kilometer race as part of my preparation and tried to forget I ran thirty plus kilometers before hitting the last ten.

I also was purposely lost in my thoughts to take away from the excruciating pain that was coming over my body. My pace was almost a walk but with a running motion.

"Left arm with right leg, right arm with left leg."

I was breaking down my strides like how Lou my physiotherapist at the Gorge Rehab Hospital taught me when I first relearned how to walk.

Having the ability to walk taken away and then gaining it back was the major reason why I wanted to do this. I also did it for those who could not due to circumstances they could not control. I was thinking of Bob and Sharon, my two angels who I met through my rehab experience. They would be so proud. I wish they were here.

I thought of Allison and the love and assistance she gave me. I have not had communiqué with her for almost four years and still have not to the present. I pray she is doing well.

I also thought of my grandmother, Winifred, who succumbed to her courageous battle with cancer two years earlier. I thought of my stepfather Brian's sister, Mary Louise who I viewed and called my aunt who also succumbed to cancer. I thought of Vincent the first person I volunteered with after my brain injury, who by volunteering with him verified my purpose.

"Awesome, Greg. Love you!"

I looked up to my right and saw it was my mother yelling those encouraging words. She and Brian were on top of an incline in the parking lot of a coffee shop as I ran underneath them on the sidewalk.

"Keep on going, son," Brian my stepfather added.

My mother then spoke to Brian asking, "Why won't he stop?" as my labored run was simply to keep me vertical.

Brian did not answer as tears rolled down his face.

The cheers of mom and Brian made me fight through the pain. I now had another two reminders of the caring and supportive people involved in my recovery from traumatic brain injury to keep going. I pressed on saying to myself over and over till I crossed the finish line.

"Allison, Winnie, Bob, Sharon, Vincent, and Mary-Louise."

Saying those six names took my pain away. As I continued to repeat them, I got stronger and the unbearable pain was easier to take.

4 Hours : 37 Minutes : 18 Seconds

Openness

I had graduated from Sault College in January two thousand one. I did so with honors receiving my occupational therapy assistant (OTA) and physiotherapist assistant (PTA) certificate.

I received my first job as a rehabilitation therapist in Hamilton, working with the brain injury population and more specifically the behaviors brought on by the patient's brain injury.

I was nervous as it was my first job interview after my life-changing ordeal. I disclosed my own brain injury and thought this would be the best approach. My first career path was in business administration with a major in human resources and I was well aware that, when you looked at my resume, there was a three-year gap with my employment and education. I viewed these three years as employment, working towards regaining my independence as well as first-hand education on brain injury.

Being a rehab therapist, I would carry out programs prescribed by the OT, PT, SLP and behavioral therapist and monitor and collect data if a behavior occurred and from this determine what may have triggered the behavior. The behavior was usually anger and agitation and this would sometimes be unexpected and come clear out of the blue.

I received the job and learned so much from colleagues in Hamilton and was grateful that I was given the opportunity. To be honest, I was scared several times but knew another rehab therapist would have my back to assist if needed. The facility had an amazing team approach.

I also learned that having a sense of humor can be helpful in deescalating a situation as well as not talking down to a patient which can come across as judgmental.

My inpatient OT Paula in my own rehabilitation always treated me this way and if I had difficulty with a task and was becoming frustrated, she would calm me down by explaining why I was having trouble and that it was due to my brain injury. She did not 'dumb it down' either. She knew I was a college graduate and even if she had to explain things in a simpler way, it did not come across as disrespectful.

How Paula treated me had a great impact on my life as when I did go back to school to become an Occupational Therapy Assistant/Physiotherapy Assistant that in my second year I decided to focus on OT rather than PT. The majority of my classmates pursued physiotherapy but I concentrated on occupational therapy.

Through my personal experience of brain injury, I was enthralled by how the mental controlled the physical and that if the brain was damaged in a certain area, the effects would be widespread. My legs were physically able but my mind did not know how to instruct them. Through learning, remembering, and sequencing the steps involved, I was able to relearn how to walk and then run.

My educational path was decided from those initial interactions with my OT and PT when I began rehabilitation. My PT who first worked with me in the rehab hospital when I was an inpatient was amazing clinically but seemed quite cold, whereas my OT in the rehab hospital was friendly, giving off a more compassionate feel.

That first impression was magnified by my brain injury but also showed me that the smallest of things can affect the outcome of the persons we support, in not only rehabilitation but also life. In my case, four years later, I made a decision based on that first impression. If I had a better first interaction with my PT, I may have been less reluctant to pursue an assistant job in physiotherapy.

This showed me, as a clinician, how we interact with those we support can have an everlasting impact. Paula treating me with dignity and respect affected my decision many years later.

After several months of working in Hamilton, I had an interview at a large rehab center in Toronto. The center was looking for a full-time occupational therapist assistant (OTA) for the summer months to help with coverage for vacationing OTs and OTAs. Similar to Hamilton, I disclosed my brain injury and was honest and up front with how this affected me and directed me to help others.

The three members on the interview panel were willing to give me a chance for summer coverage, working full time. I accepted and became an OTA working not only with the brain injury population but also with other populations, from Cardio Vascular Accidents (stroke) to those affected by aging (falls and dementia). I also would modify wheelchairs for those who required them. This would be a learning experience as I was not the best with putting things mechanically together but would learn.

I worked as hard as I could over those three months and was offered a full-time permanent position as an occupational therapy assistant at the end of my summer contract.

Before my injury and most importantly, me finding God and having a relationship with Him, if someone said "Greg, we have a job opportunity in Toronto for you," I would have not taken the job. I was fearful of the big city and something happening to me.

I did have a horrific event occur to me, but from this I was not fearful or worried as I knew God now had my back. He always did but I did not realize this.

CHAPTER TEN

Calling

It was November 10th, my five-year anniversary of my assault and when I became a person with a brain injury. I was at work which in itself was miraculous. To think I went from being unable to walk or write to even expressing my emotions to now working in the rehabilitation of others who were experiencing the same.

I viewed November 10th as my new birthday as I was in essence reborn and I wanted to celebrate and appreciate those who helped me grow up again. The four years previously, I did this as well, getting together with friends and family to celebrate how far I had come.

I would call those brought into my life by my brain injury and talk to them, thanking them for being there and how I would not forget what they had done. I would call Bob and those out west who were so instrumental in me being where I was at. Being alone in Toronto this year, I called all my family members and thanked them.

My talk with my dad was short as he did not like this anniversary and I understood his reasoning. Why would he celebrate almost losing a son to a violent assault?

My mom and Brian were present for my previous four anniversaries and saw my recovery and watched me progress with amazement. They were more accepting of my new birthday and this was also a testament to their strong faith. The three of us knew how instrumental God was in my rehabilitation and now in guiding my life to help others. In the spring, I had been baptized again for this reason.

I was baptized when I was a baby but now I understood what it meant. It was symbolic of the relationship I had with Christ and was my way of letting Him know I was following Him.

I know scripture has writings of when one should be baptized and is interpreted in different ways from denomination to denomination. The way I viewed this was as a baby we cannot comprehend how to go to the bathroom let alone the belief in a higher power. And the God I believed in would not deny an innocent baby who has not yet had holy water sprinkled on its head entry into heaven.

If I have children, I will have them blessed at my church but, as they got older and developed the ability to understand God, I would share not only my story but also the story of Jesus Christ and influence them by my actions, His actions.

I am not ignorant in that I may not be as spiritual and celebratory if I did not have the recovery I had and my brain injury left me with greater deficits physically and cognitively. Working in Hamilton and then Toronto with other persons with a brain injury and them being left with life-changing deficits did give me a sense of great guilt.

Since I was at work and had not developed friendships in Toronto as I was new to the city and by myself, to celebrate, I would provide a pizza lunch to my colleagues. The occupational therapy department knew of my history and I didn't see a problem with sharing with those who did not. My brain injury resulted in my job as an occupational therapy assistant and is part of who I am.

I sent an email on November 3rd, a week earlier and was quite vague.

"Lunch on me, in room 307. Please let me know of any allergies or any preferences, having pizza."

The lunch would be for about a dozen people, a majority being occupational therapists. As everyone gathered and the pizza was delivered, I spoke.

"Hello, as a lot of you know, I suffered a traumatic brain injury and this occurred on this day five years ago. I am very blessed with the recovery I had and now I have the opportunity to work with great people like you."

I received applause and thank you from all that attended. I sat back with a slice of pizza and a glass of pop and took it all in. I reflected on what had happened to me and was mystified. My story could only be explained by the intervention of a higher power, God.

Connection

Activities of daily life (ADL) seem so easy. Start your day off with a shower, get dressed and then head off to work. When you suffer a brain injury, what seemed to be a simple and redundant act every morning can now be extremely complicated. Complications created by the physical and cognitive impairments brought on by brain injury.

I enjoyed the therapeutic aspect of ADLs, specifically shower and dressing. This activity encompassed all aspects of rehabilitation. Speech: communicating needs, physiotherapy: transferring from a wheelchair to a bath bench in a bath tub, occupational therapy: sequencing and following a plan. To me, this was the foundation of occupational therapy. ADLs were instrumental in determining someone's basic function. As an assistant, the OT would do two showers a week with the patient and me doing one.

I was beginning an ADL program with Peter, a young man who had a brain injury from a fall. This was Peter's second stay and attempt at intense rehab as the previous time he was not ready and unable to participate. Peter had been in the system for three years and became dependent on others, especially when he was in long term care (LTC). LTC being not rehab focused due to fewer therapists and staff. With staff unable to give proper time for ADLs due to large caseloads, the staff did a majority of the shower and dressing for their residents.

I had observed the OT do the routine with Peter and then the OT observed me to make sure I followed the program with consistency. Consistency was important for someone with memory issues and with this repetition would hopefully help in remembering the routine.

"Morning, Peter," I said.

He responded with a grunt.

"Time to get up and have a shower. We will do what we did the other day."

I would assist Peter in getting into his wheelchair and we would go to the tub room where there was a bathtub with a bath bench set in the center of the tub. We would transfer onto the bath bench and he would sit and control the taps for the shower and use a handheld detachable shower head.

Peter suffered from ataxia which was sudden and sporadic muscle movements which caused involuntary twitching and this seemed to increase when concentration was required for tasks. I would let Peter struggle and would assist when a task would be leading to no success and subsequent frustration and anger.

The ADL process took time with Peter and the floor we worked on had two bathtubs for 30 patients so line ups would start to form with patients with nursing and OTs and the 'chirping' at me would start.

"How much longer, Greg?", "Why are you taking so long?" and "Others need to use it too."

I wanted Peter to do things on his own and this took longer, but dealing with the time constraints of others and explaining the rehab aspect to staff was wearing thin.

My shift began at 8:00 am but I decided from now on when I had ADLs with Peter, I would come in at 7:00 am. Peter viewed me as his arch nemesis initially. I would get him to do new tasks as he progressed, which was met sometimes with explicit language directed at me.

Before I woke him for his shower, I quietly set his toothbrush with toothpaste on the brush at his bedside sink. When we returned from the bathtub, I stopped him as he went by his sink.

"What is this?" Peter questioned as he noticed the toothbrush.

"You are going to brush your teeth," I said.

"What, f--- that!"

Peter was getting slightly annoyed with the idea.

"You want your teeth cleaned correct. I am not doing it so that leaves you Peter. You just did a majority of your shower independently, so brushing your teeth should be easy and I think you can do it."

It was not easy, but Peter persevered with intermittent cursing at himself and me. Observing his struggle, I recalled when my mom set me up the same way to brush my teeth. I did not have ataxia like Peter but at the time had severe left neglect. Being right hand dominant did not help the situation, but my mother allowed me to struggle and find items on my left, incorporating me to use my left arm and hand. My mother was teaching me independence, but we had no way of predicting I would be using this in my profession eight years later.

Peter and I worked hard together for the next month and he became independent with his ADLs. He was being discharged to LTC for a short time as his home was being modified to meet his needs. We had a meeting with the team Peter would be working with at LTC and I told them his routine and how he had carried it out on his own. There were about 12 people, including his parents, around the table with Peter. I then spoke to him and became emotional.

"Peter I don't want you to let others do things for you that you can do yourself. You proved it to me, now prove it to them."

I was worried Peter would fall back into bad habits letting others do what he could do mostly because of the system and people not having the time.

"I will," Peter replied.

Peter showed me physical limitations could be overcome and was an inspiration to me, observing him struggle doing tasks that I took for granted. I hoped he continued to fight for his independence in LTC. He could show not only the staff but also other persons with a brain injury that they too can achieve a great quality of life.

I wanted him to fight on and have as much of what I had in my recovery. I knew he had a tougher fight and pray he will.

Willing

I received a promotion four years into my occupational therapy assistant career and became a rehabilitation therapist. This was similar to my first job in health care as rehabilitation therapist in Hamilton. I loved being an occupational therapist assistant, but my promotion allowed me not only to continue work with occupational therapists but also work with physiotherapists, speech + language pathologists and behavior therapists, carrying out their programs. Also living in Toronto the pay hike was a bonus.

I would still carry out ADLs with patients with my new position and, over my four years, I saw a change in occupational therapy, especially with the frequency of ADLs being carried out. When I started, I would do an ADL once a week, with the OT doing it twice. This also lessened the burden on nursing.

"Hey, Duke," Jim spoke.

Duke was the nickname Jim gave me and a reference to John Wayne.

Was a funny nickname as I had a deep voice and would stand in the light of Jim's doorway in the morning. Funnier in that I am 5 foot 7 and small compared to Jim who was a large, middle-aged man, about 6-5' and well over 200 lbs.

I would do showering and dressing with him in the morning and we would do other occupational therapy and physiotherapy prescribed treatment programs together. We connected right away.

Others were intimidated by Jim, but I wasn't and therefore worked a lot with him. This being the reason the OT pulled back from him and passed the ADLs on to me. This and he made an inappropriate remark towards her.

Disinhibition is part of brain injury and losing that filter made you say things that you should not. I viewed this as part of brain injury and, if you dealt with the inappropriate comments in the moment, the patient would more than likely stop.

I found this happening with greater frequency with the newer and younger therapists, the next generation. Avoiding tedious work was becoming the norm. What was bothersome to me was this tedious work was more functional, meaningful, and beneficial for the patient. Doing a pen and paper task and finding 'Waldo' to me was not as an important as being able to shower, cook a meal, and navigate public transportation.

Jim's intimidation and comments did not bug me, and I viewed him as a gentle giant. He also was very intelligent, funny, and an author like me. We would chat about our histories and I was fascinated by his.

How he tried out for the Boston Bruins professional hockey team back in the day when there was only six teams and these teams would have open tryouts in communities across Canada. Jim cracked me up when he described his tryout and how he was body-checked extremely hard by a veteran hard-nosed player and in that moment said to himself, "No more hockey for me."

I was giving a talk to the patients and their families and asked Jim if he would like to come. I told him it may be repetitive as I had shared my story of brain injury with Jim and his very supportive wife Margaret.

I gave them a copy of my book as Margaret reminded me of my mom in the care she provided to Jim. One of my better friends and colleagues would get frustrated with me as I gave away my books more than sold them, even when the person receiving them offered to purchase.

My Invisible Disability was a way to educate others on brain injury rehabilitation and giving the books to those who were experiencing brain injury gave them hope and knowledge that they were not alone.

When my book was first released, I was excited that I would make millions but my editor brought me back to reality. My editor stated my book would open doors to other opportunities, like speaking and educating, and my book did exactly that. ***My Invisible Disability*** is my legacy and will be there for others when I am long gone which, to me, is amazing.

My talk followed the outline of a basic presentation: an intro, my history before my brain injury, my brain injury and rehabilitation, and ended with where I am at today. My talk like my book is very intimate and I sometimes wondered if too personal as anyone could now read it. But to me, this is how I connected with people.

The talk was well received and at the end Jim raised his hand to speak.

"You have a question, Jim?" I asked.

"No, just something I want to say. Thanks for sharing your story with us and working with you is an inspiration. And thanks for being a friend."

I was very touched by Jim's comment and was saddened by my two-word response – "You're welcome."

The patient-professional policy, keeping only a work relationship and setting boundaries with those you rehabilitated, which I had to adhere to, restricted me in my response. This baffled me as I was now part of Jim's life and brought into his life through unspeakable tribulation and when he was in a most vulnerable state.

And I completed intimate tasks with Jim, like showering and taking him to the washroom, both involving nudity. I don't think Jim, a big and strong man, ever wanted a stranger completing these most intimate tasks with him. So it bothered me when I could not respond with

"Jim, thank you for inspiring me and being my friend."

I was placed and you could even say forced into Jim's life and was supposed to not let him get close to me even though I was close to him in ways few in his life ever were. I found not forming bonds with those I worked with difficult due to this. I know the policies were set in place to protect us and the patients from getting close and to set boundaries, but circumstances beyond one's control sometimes did not allow this.

I may have misinterpreted these policies and wondered if they took into account the activities I did with Jim. I would later learn that the policies did evolve and allowed for you to use your clinical judgement when forming bonds with those you supported. This provided optimal patient first care. The presentation was also in front of some of my colleagues and I did not know how they interpreted these policies and acknowledging Jim as a friend may have led to trouble depending on their interpretation.

After Jim was discharged, we kept in contact. He and Margaret happened to live near me and we would 'run into' one another in our neighborhood and have lunch or a coffee. I now have been friends with Jim and Margret for years and see them more often as Jim is helping me with editing my second book.

I know I had to use caution and there was a chance I went beyond the patient-professional policies set by our hospital but a horrible occurrence brought Jim into one and I helped him rehabilitate from this and in the process formed a bond with him, gaining a friend.

I watched Jim with Margaret and other families supporting their loved ones and thought of how my mother supported me through my rehabilitation. I helped people for a living but always wondered if I could support my family like mom did with me and how Margaret did with Jim. I am fortunate and blessed that I have not been put in that situation.

Book Two

HEALTH CARE & HORRORS

"Even though I walk through the darkest valley, I will fear no evil, for you are with me; your rod and your staff, they comfort me."

Psalms 23:4(New International Version)[1]

1 THE HOLY BIBLE, NEW INTERNATIONAL VERSION®, NIV® Copyright © 1973, 1978, 1984, 2011 by Biblica, Inc. ® Used by permission. All rights reserved worldwide.

CHAPTER ELEVEN

Bachelors

Thanksgiving and holidays became difficult when I was thirteen. My parents separated a year earlier and the divorce was finalized when I started grade ten.

I have two sisters, one older – Kim, and one younger – Melissa, and an older brother –Scott. So, it was decided the boys stayed with dad in Sault Ste. Marie (the Soo), Ontario and the girls moved with mom to Windsor, Ontario; a five-hour plus drive away driving through Michigan.

My youngest sister Melissa was seven years old when mom, her and Kim moved to Windsor. I still have that image of saying good bye to mom and Melissa and watching them walk off, Melissa skipping while holding mom's hand.

Those initial years were hard as I missed mom and during the holidays was torn between two sides when mom and my sisters would come to the Soo for the holidays to see Scott and me, as well as my grandparents and aunt. It meant two dinners and being careful not to upset either one of my parents by not giving both sides equal time, a heavy burden for a teenager.

When I entered grade twelve, my brother moved to Windsor and lived with mom and my sisters, which meant it was just dad and I for two years. Those late teenage years were not the greatest as most of my classmates did not have the responsibilities I had and I missed out on some functions that went on during this fun part of life before it turned serious with studies at college or university.

My dad owned a restaurant and worked from six in the morning to six at night every day and even sometimes till close, which was nine o'clock.

Dad got me my first job at a department store in the mall his restaurant was located in so the nights I worked I would have dinner there and the other nights I would fend for myself or we would share cooking duties for dinners at home.

Back in the late eighties, having the choice of healthy options for dinner was not available and not a priority, resulting in me using a can opener frequently or using the oven following cooking instructions found on the back of a frozen dinner or pizza box. I bought my lunches at the school cafeteria as dad gave me more than sufficient amounts of money to purchase them as he did not have time to make them.

My friends were envious at me buying fries and gravy, burgers, or macaroni and cheese, washing them down sometimes with not one but two sodas. They did not know my circumstances and I did not share it with them. They did not know I was envious of their mother made lunches or leftovers from the family dinner table the night before.

My weight went from one hundred and sixty pounds to over two hundred in just over two years. My dad did the opposite. Being a business owner, he never had time to eat, even though he ironically owned a restaurant. Seeing dad at work, he was always on the go and when he did have time for a quick break, he never ate, having a cup of coffee in his hand and a burning cigarette in his mouth.

He would go through almost two packs of smokes a day. I remember having my dinner at the restaurant and looking at the patrons, out of forty, I would say twenty-five had a cigarette burning. A sign of the times, and I would say I second hand smoked half a pack a day back then.

I also would do our laundry, which was sometimes annoying as dad and I, as well as Scott before he moved to Windsor lived in a small two-bedroom apartment after our house was sold, so fighting other tenants for a washer or dryer was always a treat. A break from homework to see if your clothes were stolen was always interesting.

I get emotional thinking of dad and me during those two years. There was no time for father-son bonding or affection. We were products of our environment and situation. Dad would come home after working a fifteen-hour shift, lie on the couch, ask me to take off his socks and for a blanket and within minutes begin to snore.

Dad was enveloped by stress and bitterness, the dysfunction in his family caused three of his children to be in a different city. He had taken pride in us, always wanting us to have the best at his expense. Dad put Scott and me through hockey till we were eighteen which was not cheap. When you start a sport young, you grow out of your equipment quickly meaning new equipment had to be purchased.

The Soo is a small city and I know dad's pride took a huge blow with his failed marriage. He turned his focus to his restaurant and when the economy took a downward turn, dad's stress would ratchet up.

Several years later, I would go to Pembroke, Ontario, a city of just over thirteen thousand people. My father was born and raised just outside of Pembroke, two plus miles back in the bush. I went with him and two of his brothers to this small dilapidated three-bedroom house with no electricity or access to roads. My dad has three brothers and four sisters, and along with his parents and an older blind tenant, who assisted financially with rent, resided there. My father had lost two other brothers to disease. Thirteen people lived there at one point.

I would hear tales from my aunts and uncles over time about this life: walking miles to the lake for water, when the chicken stopped laying eggs, it would be in the pot the next day for dinner. It was a lifestyle of survival, no time for hugs or affection. Dad lost his father early in his life, and my grandma met someone else, his main selling point was he had a car.

I also imagined the fear of being alone with this upbringing. Dad was from a huge family but the long quiet days and nights when everyone separated to do chores. My grandfather was a lumberjack and would leave for weeks at a time. Dad must have thought 'Will I ever see him again?'

When I graduated high school, I moved to Windsor to go to university, meaning dad was on his own. He did however meet and began to date an amazing woman, Cathy. I am so grateful for this, I did not want dad to feel abandoned.

Beginning

Thanksgiving fell earlier in the calendar in two thousand and twelve. I had driven eight hours to the Soo from Toronto. Over the years with us kids becoming adults, the separate dinners over the holidays became less tense. They actually became enjoyable.

My dad married Cathy in nineteen ninety seven; my mom married her high school sweetheart Brian in nineteen ninety six. I was very blessed; I went from one parent in my teenage years to having four great ones in my adulthood.

I would refer to Brian as Pa number two and Cathy as Ma number two. I also gained eight more siblings as my new parents each had four kids of their own from their previous marriage.

This thanksgiving I would spend dinner with mom and Brian, and then go to the house of Cathy's son Kevin for dessert. I became close to Kevin as, for the past three years, we would go hiking and snowshoeing for hours over the Christmas holidays. A tradition I enjoyed, and what a cardiovascular workout.

Cathy was out west in Vancouver on vacation with her sister so it was just dad. I would visit dad more than just for dessert, I was up in the Soo for three days and being a small city him and mom were a five-minute drive away from each other.

I also wanted to check in on him. Cathy was reluctant to go on vacation due to dad's ongoing health issues. He was diabetic and suffered from Chronic Obstructive Pulmonary Disorder (COPD) which affected his breathing and he was very fatigued by the slightest of physical activity. Dad had quit smoking five years earlier, something we were all shocked by and proud of. To quit an addictive habit of almost fifty years told me of my dad's strength and will.

He also developed a persistent cough. The cough would subside at times but was always present for the past several months. Dad wanted Cathy to go on her planned vacation and told her not to worry. He also did not want any attention or fuss brought on to him.

Dad was of the mindset if you do not know what is wrong it will go away. But I noticed a rapid decline in my father. I would take two weeks off every summer and visit the Soo and over the past couple years, things started to drastically change. Two years ago, we went golfing; last year, we went to my brother's camp (northern Ontario term for cottage) and he was winded just walking the short trail in and out of the camp. This year, dad treated me to his favorite, prime rib, at the country club we used to golf at.

The dinner upset me as dad struggled through, that cough never stopped but he continued on like nothing was wrong and for this not to ruin our dinner. I would look at Cathy when dad coughed and our eyes both began to well up with tears but made sure to wipe and not let dad notice for he would get angered by this.

I had a great turkey dinner with mom and Brian and then went to Kevin's for dessert. It was a large family gathering and dad was very quiet. My father owned a room like this with funny stories and anecdotes. Something he passed on to all of his kids. I have the gift of gab and even have a habit of repeating stories like dad as I got older.

I always was amused when being first at a family function when dad was present, you would hear the same story with each new arrival. The thing was it never got old and dad's story telling improved with each rendition.

When dessert was over and after dad and I said our good byes to our extended family, we walked to our cars together.

"Starting out early tomorrow?" dad asked.

"Yep, long old drive and don't want to hit Toronto traffic at rush hour."

We came to dad's car and we usually shook hands and went our separate ways. This time dad gave me a hug. I obliged and the hug was strong and tight.

"Love you, dad."

"Love you too," dad said.

I walked to my car and realized that was the first hug dad initiated since I visited him for the first time after my assault. Dad loved us kids but did not express it much physically, especially to us boys. It was implied but was nice to feel or hear. For the year after my assault, we would say love you back and forth to each other when we conversed over the phone but once I was in the 'clear', it went away. Same with my brother, as Scott was blunter, stating, "Okay enough, I know."

The drive home the next morning was long. I had dad's hug on my mind and did not have to be a genius to know something was wrong. When I got home, I had to do my usual call to dad so he would know I made it home safe.

"Hey, dad; home."

"Great, you made pretty good time."

Dad was always concerned about making good time when we travelled on family vacations.

"Love ya, dad."

"Kay gotta go," his voice affected by his cough.

No Wind

Dad had an appointment with his doctor on November thirteenth. He had numerous tests done and a CAT scan over the weeks after thanksgiving. My brother and sisters and I were all nervous about this appointment and any news from it. Dad's deterioration was on all our minds.

I finished at work and decided to walk home, which took me about an hour and half. The walk allowed me to decompress from my day, which can be taxing sometimes as rehabilitating persons who went through what I did, brain injury, and them not having the same outcome as I wore on me.

I was entering my fifteenth year of working in some capacity,counting my volunteer work six months post my brain injury, with fellow persons with a brain injury. I had taken a year leave of absence to regroup and get a handle on how to cope with the thoughts of those less fortunate with their recovery than me in two thousand and seven. I continued to work in long term care for this year which, looking back, was maybe not the best thing to be doing considering why I took the leave in the first place.

This walk, my thoughts focused on what may lay ahead for dad. Working in health care, I was privy to what caused bad health and I knew my dad was not a great picture of health over the years. All the stress over his life, poor eating habits, rye whiskey with cola and smoking all contributed to dad's picture.

Cathy, Ma #2, would try her hardest over the years to help dad with his diet and the importance of quitting smoking and the impact the two had on him. She succeeded with the smoking and would give dad healthy meals, but he always would avoid the greens and love desserts and salty/ sweet snacks. He had an affection for chocolate bars and Pepsi Cola.

I remember lecturing my dad about diabetes over the phone and how I saw people lose limbs from the disease and reminded him how grandma, his mom, went blind from it. In one ear and out the other as we ended our conversation with our goodbyes and me asking, "What you up to tonight?"

"Making my homemade cinnamon buns," he would reply, not seeing the irony of such a response after my lecture.

I was about forty-five minutes into my walk when my cell phone vibrated. I took it out of my pocket and saw that it was my older sister Kim from Windsor. I let it ring four times; on ring five, my phone would take a message. I took a deep breath and answered.

"Hey, Kim."

There was a pause and she delivered the news.

"Dad has lung cancer," my sister said.

It was news I sadly expected, all the signs pointed to this, but it felt like my heart was being squeezed by a vice.

Both our voices were affected by emotion as we continued our conversation.

"They found a tumor about the size of a grapefruit in one of his lungs," Kim stated.

"What is the course of action? What is next?" I asked.

"Don't know yet. Dad having COPD is concerning as surgery for removal or a lung transplant is not possible."

"How is Cathy?" I questioned.

Not the smartest question but hearing your father has lung cancer and is inoperable makes you ask questions that have obvious answers.

"Upset. But we will be there for her."

"For sure we will. I am just walking home so gonna let you go sis. Love you."

"Love you too."

I got home and, after touching base with Cathy, dad was not in the mood to talk, and my other siblings and mother I laid in bed, staring at the ceiling. Before I knew it, I was on the subway going back to work. I told my colleagues when I arrived, explaining my sullen mood, and they were saddened and would lend their support whenever I needed it.

I had a research meeting at lunch. I had been working with an amazing doctor and team on a study for the past two years that looked at the impact of intense rehabilitation early on with those who suffered a severe traumatic brain injury. Instead of three to four hours of rehab, the study participant would receive six to seven, doubling the rehab they would usually receive. I was the frontline rehabilitation therapist who provided the extra hours of therapy following referrals given by the participant's team of therapists.

When I sat, one of the team members brought in a cake to celebrate my anniversary of when I received my brain injury and to commemorate how far I had come. My assault occurred on November tenth and today was the fourteenth so this beautiful act was belated because our meeting did not fall on the actual date. I was touched and moved by the thoughtful gesture. Throw in the news about dad's diagnosis the day before and I had a hard time keeping my emotions in check.

November would even get harder to forget.

CHAPTER TWELVE

Matter of Time

Two weeks had gone by and all of our families, mine and Cathy's, were trying to come to grips with dad's situation.

It was Wednesday night and I was exhausted more than usual. My fatigue, my biggest deficit from my brain injury, was in high gear. The stress of my job always had a hand in this but now that my life outside of work was lending a hand as well, it felt like I could never get enough rest as my mind was constantly racing.

I kept going with work as dad taught me my problems were not work's. He also taught me to be not only on time, but also ten minutes early wearing a pressed shirt and combed hair. Small lessons that seem to be missing from today's generation.

My father had left his tough upbringing when he was sixteen, leaving the pioneer lifestyle to manage a menswear department at a clothing store in Toronto in the early sixties. He would go on to become district manager of stores in the Ottawa area. What courage to do such a thing, leaving a place with no running water or electricity and going to the big city and making a living and excelling, making a name for yourself. Dad did not have much when he was younger and proved when given the opportunity of a great job, hard work would pay off. This way of thinking was in me as well as my brother and sisters.

I had just finished my last load of laundry and was returning to my apartment when my cell phone rang. It was Cathy.

"Hey, everything okay?" I asked.

"Your dad is in the intensive care unit (ICU). He was not feeling well and we went to emergency and now he is in ICU for monitoring," Cathy replied.

"Should I come up?" I asked.

"Don't know, Greg. It isn't good."

"I am going to get some sleep, get up early and drive up. Do not tell dad, he would worry," I said.

"Okay."

"Love you, Ma number two."

"Love you too. Careful driving."

I threw together some clothes and stuffed them in a suitcase and set my alarm for five in the morning, would not need the alarm as I did not sleep a wink. I knew cancer moved quickly but was thinking, this quick?

I began the long drive up. I made the drive part of the trip when I took my summer vacations up in the Soo. Sometimes it would take me nine hours. I would listen to music; stop for coffee a couple times as well as for lunch. Some of my friends were amazed that I would drive for so long by myself, but I enjoyed it.

This drive I focused on making great time, not too many stops or music playing to sing along to. As I approached the outskirts of the Soo, I put on Johnny Cash. It brought me back to when I was five years old. Scott was seven and Kim nine. Melissa was born seven and half years after me.

Dad had this seventy three, two door, silver Cadillac with black rag top. The car was huge and the doors were the length of two doors of today's vehicles and so heavy. You would lose your hand not just a finger if you were not paying attention when the door was closed. He would drive with mom in the front seat and us three kids in the back and we had more than ample room. The bench backseat seemed like the size of a couch.

The Caddy had an eight-track stereo and dad always had Johnny Cash playing. We would go to this outdoor diner where the menu was displayed on billboards above the diner. You would remain in the car and the waitress arrived on roller skates and took your order. We would have burgers and fries with root beer floats (root beer with a scoop of vanilla ice cream). The tray would be placed right on the rolled down window as dad gave us our meals.

I pulled up to the hospital scared and nervous of what I may see. The hospital was newer and just built and when I came to the ICU waiting room, I hit the intercom to enter, only two visitors were allowed at a time.

"Hello," the voice on the other end stated.

"Greg Noack, here to see my father Len."

There was no response but the door buzzed open for me to enter. I did not get a room number so went left around the corner. There were nurse work stations outside each of the rooms for close monitoring of the patients due to the intensive state they were in.

One workstation had an X-ray on a computer screen. The X-ray was of lungs, one lung was visible with the other gone. The X-ray looked fake, almost cartoonish, like someone held a blank white piece of paper over the missing lung. I squinted and saw a name in the right corner, L. Noack. My dad had pneumonia and his one lung filled up with fluid.

The proximity of the nurse's station told me dad was nearby. I looked in the next room I passed and there was Cathy standing at his bedside. He looked so small in that bed. He was surrounded by machines and there was a smaller machine on the floor pumping the gunk out of his one lung through a tube inserted in dad's side.

I entered the room and Cathy was surprised by my early arrival from the good time I had made on my drive, dad even more so as Cathy did not tell him as he would worry. I am glad she did not tell him as the one monitor displaying dad's heart rate showed a beats per minute of one hundred and eighty.

I was so glad I drove up; dad having COPD, one lung, and his resting heart rate remaining so high at rest I questioned how he was still alive. He was fighting cancer with all his might.

"Hey, dad."

"Hey," dad was happy to see me and what he said after did not surprise me.

"Was work okay with this?" he said.

Work would have to be as I was going to be with dad as much as I could.

My brother and sisters drove up from Windsor within hours of my arrival. Dad was not stabilizing, as his lung filled up with fluid a second time and concern was with why this was occurring.

The twelve hours or so before my siblings with their spouses and children began to arrive were taxing as I know dad was fighting for us and I was scared that once all of us were here he would pass. My mom's mother, my granny, passed away at my mother's home with mom at her side but fought until her other daughter, my aunt, was present so she could say good bye to both of her kids.

I was greedy thinking of myself, not wanting to lose my dad, not considering how he was suffering. In the moment you are not thinking straight. I had dad all my life, forty years, and the suddenness of losing him was setting in and I was not coping well.

Cathy's daughter Elaine and son Kevin with his wife Valerie, and their daughters Courtney and Carissa (both in their early twenties who dad adored and was so proud of) as well as me and another family visiting their loved one, crammed the ICU waiting room. All of us were emotional, trying to figure out what was happening with our loved one.

When it was my turn to be with dad due to the two visitors at a time rule, his resting heart rate continued to remain at one eighty. It was bothersome as you felt powerless and could do nothing. Even more so as neither did the health care team that tended to my father.

Seemed you would receive different information from different people: from the oncologist to the respiratory therapist, to the ICU doctor to different nurses who tended to dad. This confusion added to the uneasiness of the situation.

Kevin's wife Valerie was a calming influence. She works in health care and knew of all the specialists and their jobs and had a better handle on the situation. I was familiar with those involved with rehabilitation but not in acute or intensive care. Valerie knew that losing dad maybe near and helped me with the difficult calls to tell my siblings to drive up from Windsor.

My brother and sisters with their families arrived. Dad got to see us all and his lung did not fill up for a third time. He needed us all to continue his fight, and not say good bye.

Last

Dad went home after two weeks of monitoring in a general population hospital room after he had stabilized in ICU. All of us kids went home and carried on with our lives. This would be hard as we were all a five to eight-hour drive away. Knowing Cathy was there with dad as well as two of her children, Kevin and Elaine, gave us comfort.

All of us went up for Christmas except my older sister Kim, who had back surgery in two thousand and ten and had metal rods inserted into her spinal column due to a vertebra disintegrating from poor posture caused from 'wear and tear' at work. Kim was a hard worker and was a supervisor at a drug store. Kim had dad's trait of push forward no matter what when it came to work, but it came to a point where her back pain was unbearable.

In the commotion in ICU when dad had pneumonia, amongst all the information being disseminated during those anxious moments, dad's medical history was discussed. An X-ray from five years earlier was mentioned, where a spot was found on dad's lung. This was news to Cathy and all of us. Dad shielded it from us, not wanting to worry us and maybe he thought it was nothing.

This spot grew into a grapefruit size tumor that was impinging on dad's spine. Dad would receive palliative radiation and chemotherapy which would make him comfortable and this course of treatment did so for the next few months.

He also would need oxygen through a machine or from a portable tank. I hated seeing dad with those translucent prongs in his nose with the cord running across his cheeks and behind his ears. Oxygen became a permanent fixture for dad as he was functioning on one lung and along with COPD he could not produce enough oxygen on his own.

The notion avoidance and not knowing maybe the best medicine did not work for my father. I was the same way until my brain injury but after my brain injury, I made sure to have my yearly physical exam and take care of myself, my lesson was learned. I hope my brother Scott can learn from what dad was going through, to quit smoking and not follow dad. I do not want my brother to suffer like this.

Shopping for dad was extremely hard, was this going to be the last Christmas gift I would buy for him? What would I buy him? I did not what to apply too much meaning to it and cause dad to think there was no hope.

I bought him a gift certificate to his favorite Chinese buffet restaurant in the Soo and a Toronto Blue Jays baseball cap, as dad was a huge fan. He always had the Jays game on in the summer and there was a peacefulness to hearing the commentary in the background as we visited over the years.

Christmas was subdued and we would have drinks and appetizers before Christmas dinner in dad's living room. Dad always dressed up for occasions and did so for this. Nice pressed dress shirt with a dark buttoned cardigan with corduroy pants. His slippers were even dressy and coordinated well with his outfit. He sat quietly in the corner, just taking everything in.

I would look at him with those nose prongs on and became sad. My dad was not stupid. He knew the odds of winning this fight with cancer were not in his favor, especially going into the fight in bad condition.

My sadness would turn to anger as my brother would pass by dad and open the door and go outside in the freezing cold to have a smoke. What more of an example did my brother need? I looked up to my older brother and the thought of losing him possibly the same way as dad was a thought I did not want to have. Scott would quit for a while over the years and I knew he could and was strong enough to do so but would come back to the horrible habit. This showed me the powerful addiction of smoking and the hold it has on people.

Christmas and New Year's went by quickly and I wished it had gone by slower. Almost three months went by till I drove up to see dad again. It was a long weekend in March.

Maple syrup was in season at this time and the Soo area produced amazing syrup. Unlimited pancakes and sausage were offered at a cheap price at a community center near where the syrup was manufactured. It allowed you to taste the product and purchase bottles of maple syrup if you were so inclined.

Dad, Cathy, and I went, dad using a portable oxygen tank he carried. There was a lineup as we paid at the door and made our way to one of the picnic tables scattered on the floor of the center. I would go up and grab a plate for dad and myself, and would go up a couple times for us. We took advantage of the all-you-can-eat part of the deal.

We ate several portions with great amounts of syrup poured on our pancakes. In some instances, you are not concerned about being healthy with what you eat, even though this breakfast was not good for dad and his diabetes. When you are battling terminal cancer, you are more focused on quality of life. Dad liked his sweets and Cathy as well as I let him enjoy the syrup and the moment.

After many chuckles as we ate our pancakes and sausages, we went back to dad and Cathy's. We sat and visited for a bit before dad went for a sleep.

"Cathy and I want to give you something," dad said.

"Okay," I hesitantly replied.

Dad presented me with a check of great value.

"What is this for?" I questioned, becoming emotional.

"Well, Cathy and I helped your brother and sisters out on their wedding days and we want to do the same."

I was single at the time and finding a spouse was not really a priority of mine and I struggled to meet someone to share my life with over the years.

"I can't take this … you will be here on my big day, dad."

We looked at each other with a bit of a smirk when dad said, "I am not getting any younger."

I accepted the generous gift and said good bye to dad and Cathy and drove back to my mom's where I stayed. As I drove, the possibility of my father not being at my wedding or other milestones in my life was becoming a reality.

Steps back

I made the drive up to the Soo once more for the long weekend in May before my summer holidays. I spent these three days up north, mostly with dad and Cathy.

Dad and Cathy's home was a beautifully renovated one hundred year old, two story brick home that they took pride in. The Soo would have an annual beautiful Christmas lights award as well as best flower/garden award for neighborhoods. My dad and Cathy won either award on numerous occasions and later I would find out dad would call and nominate himself; calling in disguising his voice as another neighbor.

Dad and Cathy had a pullout sofa bed in their living room, which was only pulled out when needed for visitors, but now was pulled out for dad to rest. I spent a majority of my time over the three days lying beside him, talking and napping.

Working in rehab, I learned what an obstacle stairs would be as the physiotherapists and I worked on stair practice with patients so they could go home. I was startled at the high percentage of patients who would move in to a long term care facility after rehab for the reason of stairs and their home not being equipped to handle their changed selves. This was now becoming a factor for my father as his bedroom and bathroom were upstairs, a big flight of stairs consisting of two steps, a landing, then five more.

Dad would make it up the stairs to sleep at night or to use the bathroom, being sure not to get tangled in the oxygen cord that was attached to the oxygen machine that was now a permanent fixture found on the main floor. It saddened me seeing dad struggle with those stairs as he began the long difficult ascension to go to his bed or use the bathroom.

The two months after the May long weekend seemed to go by in the blink of an eye. I would talk to dad several times a week and with each conversation I heard his decline. We would discuss sports and my other siblings at length before but not anymore. My father who is such a talker and story teller and now this was even taken away from him due to insufficient oxygen.

I always chuckled when dad would call me and ask how Scott, Kim, or Melissa was and he would do the same with them, seeming not interested with the person he called.

For the past several years, I would take two weeks off in the summer and head up to the Soo and spend it with my parents. This year, I took three weeks and would spend a majority of it with dad and Cathy. My mother understood the situation and even though she and my father had their differences in the past, she was distraught by dad's diagnosis.

I needed the extra week off as dad was in ICU again due to complications and once stabilized transferred to a general hospital room. I would make the long drive up and wept openly several times. Cars that past me on the highway must have thought I was crazy but I did not care. Since my brain injury, I was more emotional but even without the effects of brain injury, I would cry. I was losing someone who I had all my life and who was part of me. My amazing colleague and doctor in research who I work with said it best, "Greg, losing a parent sucks" and "You will mourn the relationship you did not have with your father".

The latter statement made me think of my teenage years and even recently before dad became ill. Why did I not call him more or drive up more to see him? It took him dying of cancer for me to realize this and to put a greater effort forth.

I drove directly to the hospital and a deep sadness washed over me as I would turn into the laneway and look at the hospital straight ahead. Every time I drove into the parking lot and made the walk up to see dad, I was scared of what I would see.

I walked into my father's room and he had two visitors, a couple who had been friends with him for years, Don and his wife Pat. My brother Scott and Don's son played on the same hockey team when they were young.

Up in the Soo hockey was something almost every young boy played and was part of your upbringing. I was an average player, a stay at home defense man, while my brother was an excellent forward with a great mind for the game. He saw the ice differently from me, I attempted to body check everyone, handling the puck like a hot potato and Scott avoided players like me with ease. Scott was so good he was offered a walk on try out from a northern Michigan university.

While Scott and I played, our parents were in the stands watching and forming friendships. My dad and Don would stand at the glass and watch while moms would be in the stands cheering loudly. I still can recall my mom and older sister Kim being quite vocal with their cheerleading.

It was nice to see dad laughing and reminiscing, and the stories they shared made me laugh. Don and Pat said their good byes with dad saying, "When I am back on my feet, we will go out for dinner and drinks."

Don and Pat replied, 'for sure' but the reality of dad's health situation was on all our minds and forlorn faces started to creep into the room after they had left.

I sat beside dad and said, "Was nice to see them."

Dad started to weep, which I never saw from him before. I did once when I was younger when my grandma died, his mother.

"I don't want to be a burden to anyone," dad said.

"You're not, dad," I stated as I started to become emotional too.

Nothing was said for the next ten minutes or so as we composed ourselves. I really did not know what to say anyway. The most horrific thing about cancer is the hopelessness, and with it not being able to comfort your loved ones with the chance of recovery. Some patients do, but my dad's health going into his fight along with the stage and type of cancer he had showed us the writing on the wall.

"So, the physiotherapist and team say I have to walk from my bed to the door and back for me to leave," dad stated.

Dad would use a rollator, a four-wheeled walker, which would steady him and to hold if he got weak.

"We can do it," I said.

Dad then took out a small O2 saturation monitor and placed it on his finger.

I would later find out from a respected respiratory therapist I work with that the saturation monitor tells you the percentage of oxygen in your blood. For individuals with normal respiratory status, you want them greater than 95% and normally they should range between 95 and 97%. For individuals with a compromised respiratory system (i.e. COPD), you usually accept a saturation greater than 88%.

That last range would apply to my father due to his COPD but whatever specialist that dealt with dad gave him no range, maybe they had and dad forgot, and said 94%. Dad would not move until that monitor read 94%. I would also find out from my colleague that my dad's greatest addiction would now be to oxygen and his focus on the fingertip monitor was commonplace for patients like my father. I wish I had this knowledge as the months ahead and dad's obsession with that little monitor would begin to aggravate me.

After checking the monitor which read 90%, dad spoke, "We will just say I did it."

I responded with "no" and that we would continue to wait. Thirty minutes would go by with dad checking his fingertip monitor numerous times.

"What is it at?' I questioned.

"92."

"Close enough. Let's do this."

Dad responded with anger, "Got to be 94."

The therapist in me came out "Kay dad, let us just see how your O2 reacts when we move. I walk people with a rollator daily and nothing will go wrong, I will be right beside you."

With some hesitation, dad finally sat up. I put his slippers on and we did the walk. He was always looking at the monitor on his finger tip, as was I now and it improved hitting 94% as we made our way back to his bed.

"Awesome, dad, see we are good to go to get out of here tomorrow."

"Thanks, Greggy."

I made sure dad was comfortable for his night's sleep and told him I would see him at home in the morning and that I loved him.

After touching base with his nurse and reporting that we completed the walk without issue, I walked to my car. I looked to my right as I walked and saw the long term care (LTC) facility that housed almost four hundred residents and thought back to when I worked there in 2007/2008.

I never envisioned a loved one of mine having to reside in LTC but started to. Even before working in LTC, I and my siblings had made a promise that our parents would never live there.

If we could take dad home permanently, we would but this option was starting to be less viable due to the care dad needed.

After my three hours with dad, it was nice to get some fresh air.

CHAPTER THIRTEEN

Opportunities - September 28, 2007

I loosened my tie, sat on my couch and put my feet up on the coffee table in my living room. I twisted open a beer. I usually did not drink, I would have one or two socially, or to celebrate an event or occasion. Being a person with a brain injury, I knew the effects of alcohol were magnified so I usually avoided drinking.

What a Friday I had. I was the keynote speaker at a conference in Mississauga, Ontario. I spoke to health care professionals and gave my lecture in the morning. After the lecture, I drove back to Toronto, and was offered an impressive job at a national association that supported persons with paraplegia in the afternoon. I was given the weekend to think about the offer and give my decision on Monday.

I analyzed my day closely as I took a drink of my cold beverage and was astounded. The morning meant more to me, not to undervalue my amazing job offer.

I survived a horrific act of violence almost eleven years ago, suffering a traumatic brain injury, rehabilitated from this, and through my rehabilitation learned how to be a compassionate and empathetic clinician, and most importantly person. I had the experience of being on both sides, rehabilitating from brain injury and now rehabilitated others who suffered them.

The day's lecture was my biggest one yet, I have given close to twenty talks to various audiences the past six years. I never imagined my picture would be on a brochure and posters as a keynote speaker at a medical conference, let alone receive the standing ovation I did after I presented.

Not only was I moved by the standing ovation but also by Brianna, the lecturer before me who spoke on depression in the neurotrauma patient. She approached me after my lecture and we chatted. There was a break between the next series of lectures so we had time to do so.

"Greg, that was amazing," she said with tear-filled eyes.

"Thanks. I was almost incontinent emotionally from the ovation I received."

We both laughed. The term 'emotional incontinence' was something I just learned from Brianna's lecture. I have used the term 'emotionally labile' for someone who could not control their emotions. This is something I experienced firsthand in my own recovery from brain injury and with those I rehabilitated.

"I think you should give your talk to medical residents who are going to work with a neuro population," Brianna said.

"That would be awesome. Do you want to walk and talk as I have to get back to the city?" I responded.

"Sure I have to leave too."

We stood outside at our cars and discussed that state of health care. We talked about 'soft skills' such as compassion, courtesy, empathy, and treating people who we supported with respect and dignity. We were both saddened and dumbfounded that some in our profession did not have these 'soft skills'.

We exchanged our e-mail addresses and made sure to stay in contact. I felt I met Brianna for a reason and that I had another fighter to join my army against ignorance towards those with neurological trauma.

I loved giving lectures on my life-changing experience. I enjoyed giving it to health care professionals even though my seven years of working in the field revealed that you cannot teach 'soft skills'. If I could make one, if only one, health care professional look at the person they supported differently before they acted, I would feel fulfilled.

I also gave a different lecture geared to persons with a brain injury. I enjoyed giving these lectures as well, but sometimes the guilt I felt made it difficult. Looking over the audience, some of whom I personally rehabilitated, and seeing that they were not as blessed as I in their recovery wore me down. Exhaustion magnified even more due to the fatigue caused by my brain injury.

After my beer, I sprawled out on my couch and closed my eyes. I thought of my two different lectures with two different audiences and realized without one you could not have the other. I also realized a lot of my lecture was common sense, but in the health care field and sadly society, it seemed to becoming less common.

I also thought of my new job offer; if I took it, I would miss working with people like me; I was so tired.

Lost

I decided to take the amazing job offer which coordinated services for persons affected by paraplegia (as well as quadriplegia) in the Greater Toronto Area. The job was a one-year contract and the rehab facility I worked at for over six years gave me a leave of absence, meaning I could return in a year to my rehab therapist job.

This turned out to be a huge blessing as I lasted one month at the position. I knew I was in trouble when during my initial orientation and training the person I was shadowing stated that every day the job was different and he would have to deal with unique situations almost hourly.

This was not a good thing for me having suffered frontal lobe damage to my brain where a person's executive functions are located. The executive function most affected for me was organization and I became hyper organized and extremely rigid. My brain injury made me a creature of habit.

My job as a rehab therapist gave me structure and even though the hospital is a transitional facility, meaning patients on average stayed 4 to 12 weeks, I was able to develop schedules over the first week and settle in for the weeks ahead, not required to do something in the moment without preparing beforehand.

I had never given up on a job but I did not cope well in that only month and thought for my health, I had to leave. When I did talk to my manager, she suggested for me, 'Give it time and use her and others in the organization to learn the job'. I refused because I thought if the job took me another six months to learn and then in five more months my contract was up, the people we supported would suffer in those six months and it would not be fair to them. And there was a chance I could never get the hang of it. The manager was impressed by my honesty and wished me well.

I had accepted the job as I needed a break from my rehab therapist job working with the brain injury population. Rehabilitating people who suffered equal to or less trauma to their brain than me and them being left with greater deficits, physically and cognitively, wore on me. I had everything taken away from me and then given back and seeing others not have the same recovery made me question why I was so fortunate.

I also was affected by the finality of spinal cord injuries. With brain injury, there was a chance, especially in that first three to six months of recovery, to return to a similar quality of life before your injury.

In that month, I did gain a great appreciation and respect for the staff and the amazing work they did, one in particular who was in a wheelchair having suffered a spinal cord injury. I had lunch with him and other staff and he would tell of his worldly travels including deep sea diving.

I was impressed and in awe as he did more than me, an able-bodied person. When my face expressed amazement over his adventures, he acted surprised and, in the process, opened my eyes.

"Not a big deal, Greg. Why would it be?"

"I don't know…." I was struggling with my response.

"This wheelchair will never limit me. I am a person first, a person with quadriplegia."

From that point on, I made the conscious effort never to let a person's condition, be it paraplegia, brain injury, or disease, define and limit who they are. They are all people first.

I was about to meet another person with quadriplegia who was going to reiterate this.

Home

I talked to my manager at the rehab hospital and she said I was more than welcome to come back to my rehab therapist position right away. I decided not to and with her approval remained on my leave for another eleven months. I decided to move up north and spend time with my mother and father and try to figure out how to cope with the thoughts that were affecting me, the biggest one feeling guilt in my recovery from brain injury.

I accepted a position in Sault Ste. Marie, the 'Soo', at a long term care (LTC) facility in restorative care. The building, which housed close to four hundred residents, was only a few years old and quite nice for LTC.

As a rehab therapist, I did several transitions, taking a patient who could not live at home anymore, from rehab to LTC and this was probably the saddest part of my job. I would train the staff on transfers: physically assisting a patient from one place to another (wheelchair to bed, or wheelchair to commode/toilet) and give advice or strategies to use if the patient had any ongoing behaviors.

The thought of a young adult and seeing old photos of a fun and active life before their injury posted on the wall of their new home was hard to take, knowing a majority of their roommates were sometimes three to four times older.

One of the saddest traits of brain injury was that a person could live a long life in the impaired state they were given from their brain injury. And knowing this could have easily been me in LTC gave me a heavy heart, even though seeing the state of LTC my mother and family would never let me live there, and I would not allow them to reside there as well.

My job in the Soo was like the title, restore and maintain a person's quality of life. LTC was now the person's home so myself and two other restorative care workers would try to provide this to the residents through group exercise, individual stretching and walking programs, and applying hot packs for any stiffness or aches.

With the residence being so big, we split it into two sections, getting to half the residents on two days of the week, the other half on the other two days. This left Friday to get to any residents we missed. The job really was an eye-opener in lack of resources given to LTC and was scary knowing Canada has an aging population.

The comparison regarding workload was staggering. Four to five patients to be seen over an eight-hour shift in my rehabilitation job versus seeing twenty to thirty residents a day gave you little time to think or rest and most importantly did not allow you to build rapport with the person you were working with.

I was impressed by the other staff, nursing and personal support workers (PSW) whose jobs were not as pleasant as mine. There would be a nurse, a nurse's assistant, and two or three PSWs per thirty residents. In Toronto at the rehab hospital, it was a nurse per four patients. I know the two places had different functions in the 'system' and part of one's care but, to me, the scales were dramatically uneven.

LTC also showed me differences in how people were treated. The Canadian government had a strong least restraint policy, meaning you could not give restraints, physical or pharmaceutical, unless consent was received from family or a substitute decision maker (SDM).

The policy was needed as numerous people have lost their lives from restraints over the years. This policy was followed very strictly in Toronto and applying restraints was a last resort. With the staff (resources) available, allowing it to be a last resort was an option. In LTC, getting permission to apply a reverse seat belt to a wheelchair seemed a daily occurrence and getting consent was not difficult as telling family or an SDM that there was the risk of their loved one falling. I would give consent as well as there was not enough staff to monitor or keep an eye on my loved one.

"Hi, Shirley."

"Hi, Greg."

Shirley was a person with quadriplegia, having suffered a spinal cord injury as a teenager from a driving accident. She was in her sixties and lived her life to the fullest. She would be involved in any way she could at the LTC facility, making sure all residents were given proper care and attention.

I would stretch and do range of motion exercises for her arms and shoulders, more passively with me guiding her arms through the movement. We bonded from day one and I would make a point to be the one to do her stretching program.

Shirley enjoyed my sense of humor and I shared my life with her. Including how I met a girl in Toronto and was moving back there in September. Moving back was for my job more than anything else, but Shirley would get annoyed as the date of my return was nearing, stating adamantly "It is not going to work." with me and my new found love.

I always personalized my care but this seemed to become an anomaly. This was due to the lack of resources in LTC, therefore not enough time to build rapport/relationships. This was evident in my rehab job as well even though you did have greater time and ability to do so in comparison to LTC. This was taught in school that you should be wary of patient-professional relationships and not go beyond them. I knew this but went, what could have been interpreted by some, as beyond with Shirley.

She enjoyed her cups of tea after our stretching and when she ran out, I would spend three dollars which resulted in a month's worth of tea. I told Shirley we had to keep this quiet and that I could get in hot water, no pun intended, if the facility found out. I understood the risks of my tea purchase, this could be viewed as favoritism or could lead someone on in thinking I viewed them as more than a patient or resident of LTC.

I used my judgement while some I worked with avoided the risk. If Shirley was a young girl who I rehabilitated in Toronto and I sensed she may have feelings for me, I would not purchase tea or anything for her and would set my boundaries.

When I first started my job, I felt there was more personalization of care. The therapists I worked with used their judgement and would take risks but as the newer and younger therapists entered, personalization of care became less evident. I would sometimes get confused looks if I bought someone a coffee or treat, instead of a look of 'what a nice gesture' and 'maybe I will follow Greg's lead'.

Over analyzing, misinterpreting and placing these patient professional policies under a microscope to me caused some in the newer generation to shy away from getting close to the patients they supported.

The policies were there to protect both the patient and the professional but should not be used as a way to not get close with those you supported. By not personalizing care, both the clinician and patient lost as personalizing care in my view benefitted me, the clinician, and the patient. To me, personalizing care was the most effective way to build rapport and help patients, along with their loved ones, get through a traumatic time.

I also had to understand professionals did not have my shared experiences and if they did detach themselves from personalizing care as a way to cope and be able to work in their profession. By opening up and being real could cause them pain and I have to respect that. I do find this sad though as they could be missing out on something that can enlighten their lives and help them too. The patient-professional relationships I have had enlightened me, and I am grateful for this.

Fishermen

I was over two thirds through my year leave of absence and the May long weekend was fast approaching. I was able to get the Friday off from the LTC facility so I had four days off in a row. My dad and I planned to go visit his family in Pembroke, spending a majority of time visiting and fishing with his brothers at my one uncle's camp. My brother Scott and his friend Trevor would meet us there, them driving from Windsor.

The drive to me was the part I looked forward to the most. The drive was eight hours in duration and would be just dad and I. Other than the tumultuous time that dad and I had when we lived together when I was a teenager, we never really had quality alone time together.

The drive from the Soo to Pembroke brought back childhood memories, before Melissa my youngest sister was even born. My father would pile us into the station wagon and drive us to see his family. Making great time was of the utmost importance to dad and this trait has been passed onto to my brother but not me. Bathroom breaks would be limited and stopping for lunch and ordering food that took little time to prepare were our options.

I would chuckle, thinking back to dad being stern with the instruction of not making a noise when we drove through Sudbury, a city of about one hundred and fifty thousand people. Being quite young, I got the impression we were driving through New York City. Having lived in Toronto for the past several years and driving throughout southern Ontario, I realize dad's worry of driving through rush hour in Sudbury may have been unwarranted.

I was the driver this time and when I did travel to far places, I took my time, enjoying many coffee breaks, a nice lunch, and stopping to stretch. With me driving, the roles were now reversed and I did not stray from my taking my time approach to driving.

"Have to pee and grabbing another coffee," I stated, turning into a roadside coffee shop.

"Really," dad replied with annoyance.

"Yep. You want one?" I asked.

"Sure. Last stop, right?" dad inquired.

"Yes."

After driving for another hour, we made it to a small hamlet near my uncle's camp and pulled to the side of the road to call for more specific instructions and to let my uncle know we were close.

"Not bad time. We will say we left at 9:00," Dad said.

"What, no we didn't."

We both laughed at dad wanting to impress with the great time we made, even though the eight-hour drive took nine and half hours because of me.

The three days went by quickly with more visiting and laughter than fishing. I did however notice a change in dad, he slept a majority of the visit and did not move around a lot, staying in the camp to nap when we would venture off to fish or hike.

During my year stay in the Soo, I asked dad if he felt okay and he responded with 'No, not really'. After his response, there was dead silence and no expansion on the topic. Dad was okay feeling this way I guess. I would lecture him in my adult years on his diet due to his diabetes and Cathy and I as well as my family and Cathy's were on dad about smoking which he had stopped finally that year.

Looking back at the fishing trip and questioning my dad's health, I regret not pushing dad to get himself checked out but also knew this would be met with resistance or 'Don't worry; I will'. Dad would go for checkups but would do so alone and afterwards say he was fine. I would think to myself, 'What quack is he going to?' I did not want to be morbid but thought something had to be wrong with dad, just from his lifestyle over the years. I also knew my father did not want to burden us with anything. So, if there was bad news, he would keep this to himself.

I will always cherish my year off, the end of two thousand and seven and nine months into two thousand and eight. Even though I was disappointed in quitting a job, this disappointment allowed me to meet wonderful people like Shirley and see another aspect of life, that of LTC. Most importantly, I had a year with my dad, who I sensed I was starting to lose.

CHAPTER FOURTEEN

Once upon a time

Dad was able to go home the next day. Our one walk to and from the door of his hospital room the night before was sufficient. The talk of dad going into a long term care (LTC) facility was never discussed let alone the thought of palliative or end of life care.

Collectively as a family, we would not let dad or any family member live in LTC but palliative care was an option we may have considered but not my father. He viewed it as throwing in the towel even though cancer was breaking his body down and there was no way my father could fight back. Mentioning the word 'palliative' irritated my father.

Dad was receiving palliative chemotherapy and radiation whose purpose was to make him comfortable and control some of the pain and discomfort. Cancer was winning but now treatment was focusing on by how much and when the fight would end.

The huge decision of placing your loved one in a place other than home was pressed upon families at my job. Not so much palliative care but LTC, a facility that could handle and manage their care. Seeing Cathy with dad made me think of those families and my own family with me early on in my recovery from brain injury. My mother was adamant I would live with her, but gratefully I became independent and this never came to fruition.

If I did not recover the way I did, would I want to put such burden on my mother? Just helping Cathy with dad on my visits up north after he was diagnosed with lung cancer was exhausting. Exhaustion magnified by the fact it was your loved one and the fight to care for them. Cathy's job was twenty-four seven, as would be the families who decided not to put their loved one in LTC.

I was gaining a whole new perspective on caregiver stress and what this stress can do to the family dynamic. I now had a better understanding of why a spouse or family member would get short with or angered at their loved one who was battling brain injury or any trauma and disease that was threatening the life you once had with them.

Dad wanted a bath and wanted to do it on his own. He made it up the stairs, stopping at the landing, after the first two stairs to catch his breath. He had his oxygen on and still needed the rest break. He made it up the last five stairs with Cathy close behind.

He was reluctant for any assistance. Cathy did help dad in and out of the tub and with washing when he became short of breath. He placed his oxygen prongs back in his nostrils and made his way back to his bedroom across the hall. He wanted to dress alone so Cathy let him be.

Dad made his way down the stairs with plaid shorts and a crisp white golf shirt on, very stylish. My father was always fashionable and a few times over the past months when taking him to appointments, he did not have his usual look. I realized cancer was taking away my dad bit by bit, he could not be the person he once was, a well-dressed man with dignity who cared greatly about his appearance. My dad's energy had to be spent on fighting the disease and nothing else. He was putting a valiant effort forth but fighting against a disease which had few victors.

He was extremely tired after his shower and dressing, lying down on the pullout sofa afterwards which was now his bedroom over the past three months due to the energy needed to climb the stairs. A commode (portable toilet) was also placed near the pullout. I had walked in to dad sitting on the commode a couple times and he did not hide or was ashamed. Cathy went upstairs to clean and make sure everything was in order after dad's shower. When Cathy returned, she had tears in her eyes. I approached her as she went into the kitchen.

"Okay, Ma #2?" I asked.

"Yep, your dad left out what he would wear when his day comes," she replied.

I did not respond as I was overcome with sadness. What thoughts did dad have when he picked out a beautiful striped suit, with all accessories from cuff links to pocket square for the suit blazer. He wanted people to remember his style and not the way he looked during his illness.

Dad rested for the next few hours and our – Cathy and I – concern was that his bath and fresh dress was taking its toll on him. His appearance was great but he looked very uncomfortable.

"You feeling okay, dad?" I asked.

"Don't feel good, Greggy. Just can't catch my breath."

Dad who usually wore the heart rate and oxygen monitor on the tip of his index finger and this was his greatest focus was surprisingly not on. I grabbed it and put it on his finger.

His heart rate was quite high and his oxygen saturation percentage was very low.

"How is it?" dad questioned.

"To be honest, dad, not great," I answered.

I quickly looked at Cathy and spoke…

"Think we should head to emergency just to be safe."

"Okay," dad said.

I was surprised by dad's answer as over the past few months he would wait things out but now there was no hesitation. Dad was able to walk to the car with his portable oxygen tank on and Cathy and I put the transport wheelchair folded in the back seat. My older sister Kim bought the wheelchair a couple years earlier at a yard sale because it was such a great deal. Little did we know this would become such a valuable piece of equipment for dad.

When we made it to the hospital, I transferred dad from car to wheelchair. Physiotherapists and I practiced such transfers at work with patients. I now used this knowledge and experience with dad. I was grateful for having my job as it prepared me for not only car transfers with my father but also other situations with ailing family members.

When my grandfather became ill due to intestinal issues, I tended to him, giving him a shower and using a bath transfer bench in the bathtub for him to sit on while showering. I would cue and assist him throughout. I literally brought my work home with me. I understood the rehabilitation aspect of care but now was immersed in the acute and end-of-life care. I don't know if I understood this aspect and how it was being carried out.

Bad Actor

We checked in to emergency and were given a room, more of corner of the hall with a curtain pulled around it. After about an hour, dad had settled and nursing would monitor him till the physician arrived. Waiting was something we grew used to, and waiting for bad news was the worst kind of wait. We had been there for quite some time when I told Cathy to go home and rest until we got any news.

The emergency physician finally entered the room.

"Hi, Len."

"Hi, Doctor."

Dad and Cathy had dealt with this physician earlier but was the first time I met him. He was about ten years younger than me, had a shirt and tie on with white doctor's coat and looked like he had a role on one of the many television-based dramas that was about health care. He did not ask who I was. This, to me, was a red flag that his bedside manner could be lacking.

Did this doctor not realize that dad's illness affected me too? I was a part of dad and dad will always be a part of me.

At work I would always introduce myself to whoever was in my patient's room and discover their relation to that patient. I would easily get a sense of what this loved one was like and if they seemed down would offer to make them a beverage, be it a tea or coffee, which could be made in the lounge on the floor.

"Can you sit up, Len?" the doctor requested.

Dad did and the doctor used a stethoscope to assess dad's breathing. He placed the hearing piece on dad's upper back.

"Take a deep breath for me, Len…and another."

"How is it, doctor?" my father asked.

"Glad they are not my lungs," the doctor responded.

The expression 'if looks could kill' would be defined with a picture of my face alongside of it. I almost bit through my lip trying not to voice my utter disgust with such a response. The young doctor felt my glare following his insensitive comment with, "Relatively speaking."

I replied with, "Does not make what you said any better."

He finished up with his assessment of dad and left the room, with my always gracious father thanking him. I did not say anything and looked the other way when he left.

"Asshole," I muttered.

"Greg, he does a good job," dad said in his defense.

"Get some rest, dad. I will call Cathy."

As I sat beside dad, I was so angry by what had just happened. Dad always wanted to be courteous and he thought that if you complain the care you receive would be affected. This way of thinking did not surprise me as patients that I rehabilitated would confide their displeasure with their care to me but on the condition that it was kept between us as the thought dad had was commonplace.

As I sat there, a male nurse wandered into dad's room. Cathy had purchased the local newspaper, set it folded, and placed it on dad's bedside table. This would be for dad to read later as we would be in the room for several hours until dad stabilized. This nurse, who came in, was not assigned to dad, grabbing the paper, opening it up, and reading it leaning against the wall.

He never noticed me sitting with dad but he knew now.

"Hey!"

He slowly showed himself as the opened newspaper was lowered to reveal his face.

"Is that yours?" I questioned.

He did not respond.

"Put it down and unless you are here to take care of my father, leave."

He did just that as I listened closely, hoping for a comment. I was ready to blow and dad's situation was the dynamite with the care he was receiving the fuse. I took a deep breath and sat as dad slept.

I pondered in the several hours before dad and I were able to go home about the boundaries in health care to be aware of, both good and bad. I wondered how I could change those in the caring profession to have more compassion and be more patient and family focused. Simple things like asking how you are and not touching a personal item, even a newspaper, that are not yours.

I would attempt to do so a year later, as I lectured close to 200 medical residents who would go on to become doctors. I shared my "Glad not my lungs story." with them in the hope they would be as shocked as I was and know the importance of bedside manner.

Again, to me, this was all common sense but with dad's experience and when I returned to work, it was becoming more evident some in the health care profession needed a refresher course.

Calm before

'Dad's days were numbered and was not long for the world' something one of his brother's stated to me while visiting dad probably for his last time. It was a blunt observation but that is how my father's family were, honest and to the point. There was no sugar coating. I knew dad was beyond recovery with his cancer but still did not want to accept this or hear it.

I was heading over to see him and my little sister Melissa who with her husband Dan brought my niece Lyla up from Windsor to see dad for the first time. This was an important visit for Melissa as dad's diagnosis fell close to when she received the wonderful news she would become a mother. This was the first day of their visit and the last week of my three-week vacation before returning to Toronto.

I got drenched running to my car as the Soo was experiencing a severe thunderstorm. I was driving over to see dad, my niece and family. I wanted to stop at the grocery store and buy dad a couple things, some frozen pizza and some drumstick ice cream cones, things he loved. Not very healthy but dad was not eating much and why not let him enjoy eating when he could.

I was very wet going into the store and when I made it back to my car after, I was dripping; the storm was not letting up. As I turned the corner onto dad's street, there was an ambulance parked in front of his house with sirens on. I cursed to myself for stopping at the store and started to cry. I did not know what I was walking into but was very grateful dad got to see and hold his granddaughter.

I rushed into the front door and dad had an oxygen mask on and was placed by the two paramedics on to a gurney.

"I am here, dad," I said.

The storm had caused a power outage which stopped his oxygen tank in his house. He did have a backup portable tank but the panic of the situation caused dad's vitals to skyrocket and they were not coming down. In the chaos, dad asked to see Lyla again and she was held close to him. He rubbed her cheek and said goodbye as a tear trickled down his face.

We were all weeping which was halted when dad said one last thing, "Keep an eye on that lasagna."

Cathy had bought homemade lasagna from one of the many great Italian restaurants in the Soo. Dad was concerned with us having a great dinner and the fact this was on his mind was baffling to all of us.

Cathy went in the ambulance with dad and we would go up to the hospital shortly after. Kevin would drive with me, Melissa and Dan. Kevin's wife Val and daughter Carissa would take care of Lyla. As we began the drive, I thought of dad agreeing to sign a do not resuscitate (DNR) order, meaning not to go beyond measures to save him if the situation escalated.

I had done my placement for my rehabilitation certificate at a small eastern Ontario county hospital where I observed how a DNR could be.

I was in a four-patient room treating one of the patients when another patient lying in their bed went into convulsions. The team with doctor responded quickly and after a short period of time pulled the curtain around the bed and exited the room. I could still hear the struggle but then this subsided and was followed by silence. I found this sad as this person's last moments on this earth were horrible and experienced them alone, even though their pain was now over.

"Guys," I broke the silence of our drive to the hospital, "if it comes to the point where dad is beyond help, I will stay with dad and Cathy."

"Okay," Melissa responded.

We walked into the emergency area and checked in with the nurse who would buzz visitors in the security entrance to get to dad's room.

"All of you?" she asked abruptly.

"Yes," I snapped back.

This young nurse's attitude was something I did not have time for as my father could be dying or have passed away. To act this way, in this moment where a family member's loved one could be in deep trouble, aggravated me. We were buzzed in and walked around the corner and after a nurse had pointed out dad's room, we walked in.

Dad's vitals had settled and he stabilized, meaning he was okay for now. We were relieved and chatted for a few minutes with dad. We could not talk much as even conversation was difficult for dad and he would need oxygen to respond, something he did not have enough of at the moment.

Dad was upset as he would likely stay in the hospital for the rest of Melissa and Lyla's stay. He also asked how the lasagna was and we had to lie, saying it was great.

After we had left, the four of us stood in the hallway, exhausted by the sadness of the situation. The emergency nurse, who buzzed us in, greeting us so coldly and annoyed that she had to deal with us, walked by with a large coffee in her hand and spoke.

"Ah, you can't all stand here. Please wait outside the emergency area."

We followed her and I had to be calmed down by my sister.

"Who does this nurse think she is?"

"Greg, easy…" Melissa replied.

We sat outside in the waiting area, discussing what was next and I just sat glaring at the rude nurse who sat at her work station drinking her coffee. I did not break my glare for about a minute when Melissa told me to stop as she was even starting to feel uncomfortable. I did not listen to my sister and was happy the nurse was nervous about me. As we left, I continued to glare at her. Her behavior made me and my family uncomfortable and sadly I resorted to her level with my behavior in that

I hoped she felt uncomfortable too. I was not proud of myself, sinking to her level.

CHAPTER FIFTEEN

Hidden

Dad remained in the hospital and ICU for the rest of my vacation. Dad was correct in that he would end up not being able to be with his granddaughter. We would all go and see him numerous times but Lyla was not allowed due to those in ICU having compromised immune systems as well as Lyla being a new born.

I was not there when a lovely nurse allowed Melissa and Dan with Lyla to sneak in a backway for dad to say good bye. Melissa described the scene to me and heart-wrenching would be describing it mildly. We were blessed this nurse put the needs of her patient first so dad could see Lyla one last time.

For the remainder of my vacation, I would go up to ICU and see dad daily. In the time I was not seeing dad, I went to the gym or took time to rest and reflect on the three weeks I had spent helping with the care of my father.

I reflected on the bitterness that struck me near the end of my second week. I realized my past was subconsciously eating at me, specifically when dad left me when I almost died 17 years earlier. With discussions with mom, she calmed me down as she sensed I was teetering on the edge of voicing my displeasure from my past.

Dad could not cope with losing his son, me, and flew back east when I was in rough shape right after my traumatic brain injury. I never blamed him for this as he was a product of his upbringing, one that was strictly of survival. I also don't blame him especially now, as seeing dad dying in front of me was the most difficult thing I witnessed in my life and I now better understand his perspective as running from the situation would have caused me less pain. I would never do this because it is my dad and even though my upbringing was difficult at times, it was good with love more present in my upbringing than just survival.

I reflected on cancer and how this disgusting disease affects everyone. I know I am not the only one who thinks big pharmaceutical companies are hiding a cure. This thought was diminished when my stepbrother Kevin and I went to his in-law's cottage to get away one evening. Kevin is a high school biology teacher and very intelligent. In our conversation, I brought up the notion of drug companies holding back a cure and he replied, "That researchers and scientists still cannot determine how cancer mutates, Greg, let alone stop the disease. There is a new type of cancer found every week." I also knew with the expanse of social media if someone knew of a cure, they would break the news not being able to keep in such a revelation.

I also thought of my return to work. This would be difficult as I worked with a majority of those who cared alongside the small minority who seemed not to, similar to the health care workers who cared for my father. This minority affected me over the years but now the aggravation the few caused would be magnified with my care giving experiences with dad.

I did more self-reflection on my many years of work in health care and when I would observe subtle and not so subtle mistreatment, or in this case lack of treatment, of patients. I would get very frustrated by the select few repeat offenders who would have one-hour treatment sessions that began 10-15 minutes late of their scheduled time and would also end 10 minutes early, 'short-changing' as I liked to call this. A patient should receive that scheduled hour of therapy daily during their stay and when a therapist would short-change, the accumulative five hours for the week would be more like three hours. To expand even more, if I experienced 'short changing' when I was in rehab, which was a four-week stay, 20 hours would have been 12 hours, meaning I would have lost 40% of my expected therapy time.

I was very grateful this did not happen, and my mom and girlfriend were there to advocate for me if this did occur. But some patients do not have advocates and to make matters worse a colleague of mine once deflected their tardiness onto the patient not being able to remember using the patient's memory deficits against them.

When voicing my concerns to others who observed this as well, I would hear the response, "This happens everywhere, Greg and is sadly worse in other places." I was reluctant to believe such a statement but now after observing dad's treatment, having worked in long term care, as well as rehabilitation and from my own rehabilitation experience, this may be a systematic issue in health care.

I went up to see dad before I returned to Toronto to say good bye. I bought us coffee and really had difficulty thinking of what to talk about. Dad was limited to converse due to his lack of oxygen. We couldn't talk about sports as thoroughly as we used to or family life. Dad would always make me laugh when beginning our conversations about my other siblings with 'Not that it is any of my business'. When dad led off with this line, I knew he was looking for information on a situation. I would later give him the nickname spin doctor as he would give his opinion and state again that it was none of his business but would get things going and hear the fall out.

I was starting to get emotional as I walked to dad's room. He was still here in the flesh but I was losing the moments I took for granted earlier, the simple activity of discussing sports and family and the laughing.

Man, we had some laughs in the later years, dad was such a jokester.

I remember the first time dad took me golfing, was a par 3 course. The first hole I ever golfed I parred and dad was quite impressed, I was even more so not realizing was a simple case of beginner's luck. As we waited on the second tee off, I vigorously took practice swings while the grouping ahead of us played the hole. With the fresh dew on the grass as it was early in the morning, I slipped, throwing my legs out from underneath me with my 'expert' practice swings.

I lay on my back, looking up to the blue sky and hearing dad state, "What the heck is wrong with you? Are you okay?"

I grunted yep and we both began to laugh. I would score a seven on the hole, showing my true golf self.

"Hey, dad," I said, setting his coffee on the bedside table in front of him.

"Hate this long old drive," I added.

"Well, you better get going," dad replied.

I could see he was becoming upset and on the brink of crying. I didn't even take a sip of my coffee.

"Okay. Love you, dad and will be back up again soon."

Dad gave me an out and I used it, not staying but we were both people that sometimes ran from our emotions. I realized I was more like him than I thought. I wish I did not run away this time, as it was my last opportunity to really talk and reminisce with my father. I am going to miss him.

Friends with Benefits

My three-week vacation, using the term loosely, was exhausting and sad. I watched my father digress and almost vanish physically before my eyes and so rapidly I still had troubles grasping how a disease like this exists today.

The three weeks made me look inward, at my own work. My best and most important work was done in that three-week vacation, tending to dad. All of my work experiences from transfers, to walking patients with a walker, to using strategies to decrease my dad's agitation caused by his fear. These three weeks resulted in me viewing my colleagues differently and through a new 'lens'.

When I overheard two clinicians use the term 'a shit show' for describing a patient, I became befuddled as to what would make them use such a term. We all needed to remember that 'shit show' is someone's loved one and could be you or someone you loved.

The hierarchy that exists in health care often prevents others from speaking out, including me. For example, I work and take direction from regulated health care professionals (OT, PT, and SLP) as they provided me with treatment programs to carry out with patients. With my position not being regulated, I fell under their clinician insurance as they were regulated under a professional college. I had to follow their treatment program exactly as I was an extension of their practice.

With these working relationships, sometimes regulated staff would give off the feeling of superiority. And if I did give feedback or speak out, I know I would receive the "who are you, you are not part of our professional group" attitude. I prefer to say clique over group as if you called out one, the others would defend them even if wrong, very similar to a group of teens in high school.

This 'above you' attitude irked me as new graduates with no experience did not respect my 15 years of experience due to a piece of paper they had. I am not belittling the hard work and six years of university education they had endured and commend them for this, but respecting others' education through life and work experience should be commended as well.

Even with this childish clique environment, I never understood how you could call a patient a 'shit show'. I was curious as to what caused clinicians to behave this way. Was it the millennial mindset and with that mindset, soft skills such as compassion and empathy were decreasing?

Through my many years of employment, I heard the excuse they don't have it anymore and that they are burnt out for the health care worker who was near retirement and put in decades of exhausting, caring work. Understandable I guess but not acceptable. I have been involved in health care for over fifteen years and am exhausted but could never turn and if I sensed I was, I would leave my profession.

What bothered me was burnout was not the case. The therapists using the term were younger and new to the field. They seemed to be about themselves and getting ahead. The health care industry was like other industries in that you only thought of yourself and what was best for you and your career. This would be easier to accept in the business world where the bottom line was involved and productivity and sales were rewarded.

I was always sensitive to how persons with a brain injury were treated, especially by those who were involved with their care. I was now even more wary of the families involved as I was part of one in dealing with my father.

Over the years, I would hear the term 'difficult family' used by some clinicians, I preferred 'advocating family member'. If a family member thought their loved one was not receiving proper care or was mistreated, I did not mind if they pointed such out. I know some of my colleagues did not like this and thus the term 'difficult' was used. This also made me ponder the poor souls who did not have a family or any support to speak up for them. I am one hundred percent sure if not for my difficult mother, I would not be here today.

I do not mind saying I was difficult along with my stepmom Cathy, in the caring dad was receiving.

Having worked for over twelve years in rehabilitation, I saw a change in my work culture; this change, to me, was definitely caused by age. When I started as a therapy assistant, the therapists who I worked with were older than me with a few close to my age. I don't know if it was maturity or their own experiences, both work and personal, but I sensed greater compassion towards the patients they treated.

With my ongoing work experience and I myself getting older, I found the average age of my colleagues were anywhere from 7 to 20 years younger than me. With this, there was an immaturity to them, those cliques would form and I found performance issues were easier to ignore as you would not call out or give feedback to a friend. The old 'ignore mine and I will ignore yours' way of thinking.

This hardened me over time as the patients would suffer. If I was doing something wrong I would want to know, especially if it was to the detriment of the patient I was rehabilitating.

I thought of an incident at work which emphasized the latter.

A young man Spencer, who I worked with, was now ALC, alternate level of care. ALC occurred when the only things preventing the patient from leaving was their discharge destination, be it modifications being done to their home or a long wait for a long term care facility. The team would move on to other patients, decreasing the hours of rehab. Part of the way health care worked, prioritizing resources. ALC was also a reminder to families that they would have to soon move their loved ones elsewhere.

My job allowed me to continue on with him, maintaining what he had gained before becoming ALC. Instead of four hours of rehab a day, he would get a half hour with me daily and another hour every other day with another therapist.

I would hear not so flattering comments about Spencer near the end of his stay as he was aggressive and easily agitated but rightfully so. His life was harder to bare compared to before and I think his team forgot this and had little patience for his behaviors.

While working with him, I talked about a variety of things: my father being ill, going to the gym as he was in to working out, and my own experience with rehab from brain injury. I did not mind sharing personal items with the people I rehabilitated. It was how I connected with them. I knew not to get too personal due to patient-professional policies but allowing them to share advice and helping me made them feel good or even normal and maybe forget the situation they were in.

As we were talking, he mentioned he lost a parent to cancer and shared some insightful advice with me. He also mentioned it was his birthday.

"Happy birthday, man," I said.

"Thanks."

"What do you take in your coffee?" I questioned.

"Milk and sweetener, why?" Spencer questioned.

"Going to grab myself one and get you one too, a birthday treat," I replied.

"Thanks."

After saying bye, I went to our cafeteria which had a coffee and donut shop and purchased him a coffee and donut. Upon return, I passed through my office which also was the office for about a dozen therapists. When I did, I was met with a snide remark.

"Another coffee run?" one of the therapists who worked with Spencer stated.

"Yeah, but not for me, it is Spencer's birthday."

"Ohh…." they replied.

The therapist was hushed by my response, being a part of Spencer's team.

The next day, this therapist brought in a cake and balloons and had a get-together for Spencer in the patient dining area for all to see. Made me wonder if I did not go through that office with our coffees, would this have happened; would the therapist have put forth such an effort? I wish I did not view this gesture this way but knew some of my colleagues had ulterior motives for their actions. I was happy though for Spencer as he got attention on this day but after would be just me continuing to see him sporadically the rest of his stay.

"Thanks for having me over for dinner," I said to one of my colleagues as we walked to the planned dinner for me.

Two of my colleagues, who I communicated with when I was tending to my father up north, along with their partners, wanted to have me over for dinner.

"No problem. We were going to take you out but instead why not have a BBQ?" they inquired.

"I don't mind, don't get a chance to BBQ cause I rent, so looking forward to it."

When we arrived, the door to my colleague's home opened to about 20 of my colleagues. I was very moved by this. They organized a potluck and BBQ for me, to take my mind away from what I was going through with my dad.

This fellowship gave me hope that compassion does exist inside of my colleagues and the younger generation and that this compassion should not just be given to friends/me but those we cared for in rehab. I thanked them and had a wonderful time. As I sat and scanned the room, I thought of dad and I also thought of Spencer. Would some view my father as a 'shit show' and me advocating for him as difficult? I wish I just wore 'rose colored glasses'.

Home Stretch

My time at work after returning from my vacation I was miserable and becoming jaded. Beautiful gestures from the wonderful BBQ planned for me and the amazing work done by a majority of my colleagues I ignored. The smallest of things I observed grabbed my attention and ate at me.

From colleagues arriving and departing whenever they pleased, being late for therapy times and even shortening afternoon therapy sessions so they could leave early to go home. To even the extreme of a physiotherapist leaving a patient unattended on cardio equipment and forgetting to return to help the patient get off the machine. What bothered me is this didn't bother them in that this was the patient's only chance at rehabilitation as an inpatient, receiving intensive rehabilitation.

The magnitude of this time was crucial as it was just after the person's brain injury and that first 3-6 months is when the brain had the greatest opportunity of recovery. And with the health care system, this was your one and only chance.

I called Cathy's cellphone to talk to dad. He was home for 10 days after I had left and then was in ICU again due to more complications. He stabilized after a few days and was put in a general room and had been there for almost three weeks.

Dad was nearing the end. When Cathy put the phone up to dad for him to talk, I could not understand him. He wore an oxygen mask permanently and could only mutter small words. I then spoke to Cathy.

"How is he?" I asked, knowing the answer.

Cathy stalled with her response.

"Well..." before she finished, I said, "I will be up tomorrow by 1:00 in the afternoon."

I packed up a suitcase and put a suit in a garment bag in case it was needed. I began the long drive at 5:00 in the morning. I was lost in thought. I prepared myself on what I was going to see. I also prepared to say the hardest thing to my father. Telling him he was a great dad and that he could go. Dad was fighting for us kids and Cathy and I wanted him to know it was okay to go and that I was proud of him. I did not want him to suffer anymore.

When I entered dad's room, I was distraught. He lied in his bed supine, looking up to the ceiling, and there seemed to be nothing physically left of him. Dad and I were built the same, both short and stocky, with dad having a bigger belly than me as he got older. He was always around roughly 190 pounds but lying in that bed he looked half that.

I hugged Cathy and my cousin Ruthie, dad's niece, as she was helping with the care of dad. Ruthie and Cathy would rotate being with dad and I was grateful Ruthie did this, to lessen the burden on Cathy. This did not surprise me as Ruthie was an amazing woman who viewed dad as a father figure as she lost her dad at a younger age, my Uncle Kenny. I also connected with Ruthie on a different level as she and her husband Jack were devout Christians like me.

"Hi, Ruthie. How are you?" I asked.

"Good, Greg. Great to see you," she replied.

"Thanks for helping out and being here with dad," I stated.

"Not a problem, love Lennox."

After my eight-hour drive and thinking about it, I mustered the courage to say what I needed to dad. I leaned over him, and gently spoke.

"Dad," he looked at me with his oxygen mask on and muttered, "Yes."

I took a deep breath.

"I am so proud of you, dad. You have been a great father to me and us kids. I want you to know you can go," I said, my voice starting to break with emotion.

Dad then responded, "I am not f---ing going anywhere."

I stepped back, looking at Cathy and Ruthie, with my hand over my mouth. I did not want dad to see me cry so I left the room. Dad wanted to continue to fight, but this saddened me knowing he could not win. Cancer took everything away from dad, but he was not letting it take away his fighting spirit.

Ruthie came out in the hallway to talk to me.

"You okay?" she asked.

"I guess, just breaks my heart," I replied.

I then asked Ruthie, "Where is dad with God?"

"He is good," she responded.

Ruthie and her husband Jack lived in a small community just outside the Soo and attended a small church there. Dad did attend as well a few times over the years and bonded with the reverend, John.

I really did not know where dad stood with his relationship with God and he did not share his beliefs with me ever. But I was concerned he would not be saved when his day came.

"Do you think Reverend John could come for a visit tomorrow?" I asked.

"Sure, I will arrange it," Ruthie replied.

"Great."

A sense of relief came over me. I wanted to be sure I would see my dad again, in eternity and let dad also give some of the pain and fighting over to Christ our savior. I know my cousin Ruthie wanted the same and she knew this would put my mind at ease.

CHAPTER SIXTEEN

Found

I decided to spend the night with dad to give Cathy a break. There was a small sofa against the wall to the side of dad's bed for me to sleep on. The sofa was not long and I would be scrunched up and uncomfortable. Even if comfortable, I would not be able to sleep. Watching if dad was breathing and that he was comfortable was my job.

Cathy warned me that dad would get agitated and pull his oxygen mask off. Dad was not giving up the fight but was confused and when he felt the feeling of suffocation, he would yank the mask off to get more air. This feeling dad had for months was so horrific more so with his lifelong fear of drowning.

A friend of mine who worked at the hospital told me he popped in to see dad and that dad had pulled his mask off and his face was purple. Hearing this, I now questioned if they were checking in on him enough, they probably did but this made me anxious. Dad did not have the ability to communicate and use the call bell to prompt staff he was in distress. I later would hear that by dad being in a general hospital, staff were not trained in palliative care. Don't most hospital policies state checking in on your patients regularly not just on palliative care units?

My view was no matter what stage or level of care required, patients in hospitals should be tended to as much as resources allowed and most importantly with compassion.

Dad's state was so dire that just transferring him to palliative care and putting him on a gurney then into an ambulance would result in death. Because he digressed so rapidly, he was stuck in a place that could not care for him properly.

After dropping my suitcase off at mom's where I showered, had an early dinner and visited with her, I returned to the hospital and set up for the evening. I had my phone which had the Internet, a sports magazine, and pen and notepad as I was journaling more frequently.

When I arrived, dad needed to go to the bathroom so I stayed outside his room. I heard his nurse Thomas talking to dad and from what I heard and pieced together, dad refused a bedpan wanting to transfer to the commode chair. Thomas was reluctant as the transfer alone would use oxygen dad did not have. Thomas obliged but after the transfer, I heard Thomas almost plead with dad for a response.

"Len, Len, Mr. Noack ..."

I was waiting for Thomas to call a code blue, a call I heard at work when a patient was in extreme distress and more team assistance was required, including that of a doctor.

"Okay, Len. Okay," Thomas said with relief in his voice.

Dad was alert and was able to sit over the toilet like a normal person. I was emotional hearing the commotion as this told me two things, dad was still cognitively with us and secondly he would continue to fight for normalcy even in his state. After dad had been put in bed, I sat in a chair to the side of him.

"I am right here, dad," I spoke, leaning over to rub his arm.

He turned his head to the side to acknowledge I was there and then looked back upward. I stared at dad who lay supine with transparent oxygen mask on and this is how he was for the past month or so. I started to well up with tears looking at him, half the man he was physically, with staring towards the ceiling his only option. I was thinking what he must be thinking. Would his end be painful? When would it come?

Dad sensed my emotion even though I was trying to hide it.

He turned his head to me and spoke: "I am sorry."

When he said that, all the air in my lungs dissipated as if I was punched in the stomach. I was able to compose myself and responded.

"For what? Love you, dad and I am here for you; you're my dad."

Dad did not respond and those would be his last words he directed towards me. In the months to come, I attempted to apply meaning to what dad had meant. Was he sorry for the rough times when I was younger? Was he sorry for not being able to cope and being there for me more when I almost died? He may have been; I will never know as he did not have the ability to communicate and expand on his apology.

To me, he was sorry for putting me through the suffering he was going through and being a burden. I wish he did not feel this way because this told me dad did not realize how truly loved he was by his children.

We feared dad and his temper when growing up and his anxiety of something happening to us did not allow him to feel our love back.

I tried to get comfortable for the night and would be woken hourly by his caring young nurse Shenise, who administered dad medication to make him comfortable. I would not have slept anyway as I was thinking back on my relationship with my father. I wish I had greater discussions with dad and how I felt. Noack men shied away from our emotions and coped by not talking about things.

> "Looking unto Jesus the author and finisher of **our** faith; who for the joy that was set before him endured the cross, despising the shame, and is set down at the right hand of the throne of God."
>
> *Hebrews 12:2 (King James Version)*

At Rest

After going home and showering, resting and having lunch with my mom, I returned to see dad. Cathy and my cousin Ruth were at dad's bedside every hour if someone was not present. Dad did not have the ability to use the call bell as he just lay on his back, looking towards the ceiling and not moving.

Just leaving dad for three hours, I noticed how he deteriorated. His covered up body was getting smaller and smaller. Dad's nurse was about to give him a bed bath when I got up from sitting at his bedside and assisted her.

We would get dad to roll side to side which was more me rocking and keeping him on his side by gently pushing his shoulder forward as the nurse tended to his back and backside. The young nurse was very gentle and I decided to talk to her. The small talk was more of a distraction for me as I tried not to focus on my poor father and the state he was in.

"Nursing, respect that. I work with some amazing nurses," I said.

"Love my job but has its difficult moments," she replied.

"I am Greg by the way."

"I am Irene. Greg Noack. Heard that name before. Do you have a book?"

I was surprised by her question.

"Yes, I do."

"You talk about my step mother," Irene said.

It took a second but then clicked in.

"Carmen, correct?" I questioned.

"Yep, she married my dad and she is amazing. She had your book and is a great read. You mentioned her at the beginning."

Carmen was the first love of my life when I was a teenager and I met her at my first job. She knew dad as his restaurant was in the same mall as the department store we worked at together. We would connect over the years but with the passing of time and with life, it lessened, her getting married and having children and remaining in the Soo and me doing the opposite.

"Tell her I say hi and tell your dad he raised a lovely daughter," I said.

"Thanks."

Shortly after Irene had left, Reverend John arrived. I wanted him to talk to dad and let him know Christ would take away his suffering and his sin and this would give him peace as well as me. I wanted dad to be in heaven and live in its graces for eternity and by believing in Christ as his savior, he would have this and I also would see him again when I die.

Being a born again Christian, I always was reluctant to share my beliefs and failed with the evangelical aspect of my faith. I found Toronto with its political correctness that I was always afraid of offending someone whose beliefs were different from mine.

The way I looked at it why not believe; a belief in someone that makes you a better human being. And when judgement comes, if there is one, and I am wrong, so be it. I know it sets my mind at ease while I am alive that I will see my loved ones again so why not believe? Dad rarely went to church but, when he did, he liked Reverend John. I chuckle at the joke my father told to him.

A man was picking blueberries when a large black bear noticed him and gave chase. The blueberry picker started to run and tripped and fell and laid on his back. He knew he was done for. So, he closed his eyes and prayed, asking that the bear be a Christian and not to attack him. As he lay there, eyes closed for what seemed forever as the bear stood above him, he pondered what was taking the bear so long. He opened his eyes and saw the bear looking skyward and saying a prayer of his own.

"Thank you Lord for this meal I am about to eat."

Only my father would tell a joke to a reverend to break the ice.

"Nice to meet you, sir. I am Greg, Len's son," I spoke, shaking the reverend's hand.

"Nice to meet you," the reverend said and then hugged Cathy and my cousin Ruth.

"Good to see you, Lennox," Reverend John said as he spoke to dad at the foot of his bed.

My father said, "Hi, Reverend." which was muffled by the oxygen mask and condition he was in. I almost started to cry as my father was still 'with it' as cancer ravaged everything but his cognition.

As we sat, I asked Reverend John, "Is dad good with God."

"Your father is very quiet about his faith but he is a 316er. He believes God gave his Son and he believes this and in Him and therefore will live beyond here and for eternity."

Dad was like me in that we didn't talk about our faith and we kept quiet when amongst others who did not share the same beliefs. I was relieved that he was a believer but also was saddened that we kept this quiet amongst ourselves, missing out on sharing our faith. My father was about to be born again.

The Right to Fight

The night I had with dad was the worst night of my life. Watching him fight for his and observing the treatment given from his nurse was overwhelming. Cathy came in to relieve me so I could go to mom's to grab a bite to eat, shower, and rest for a bit.

"How was the night?" Cathy questioned.

"Not good, his nurse was horrible and dad suffered."

Cathy wasn't surprised as when she left the previous night she sensed it would be a long one as the nurse began his shift and displayed no empathy to dad and I's situation. Just how he interacted with dad from the start showed he did not care and was there for the paycheck. His actions really impacted me and Cathy as dad's last moments were fleeting and they were spent with this nurse.

The palliative doctor entered the room and said hi to dad. Dad surprisingly responded with 'How are you, doctor?'

The palliative doctor also was my dad's family doctor. He was taken aback by the appearance of dad and turned to me and Cathy.

"How was his night?" the doctor asked.

I shook my head and said, "Not good." This was difficult to say as dad lay right beside me as I answered.

The doctor knew dad was not well and asked Cathy permission to increase certain medications but with these increases, we would be saying good bye to him. By making dad comfortable, we would be losing him. Cathy and I looked at each other and nodded in agreement and Cathy said yes to the increase in dosage.

Once the doctor left, I said bye to Cathy and dad, saying I loved him and would be back in the afternoon. This would be the last time dad would hear and understand my words.

As I walked to my car, I called my brother in Windsor. He answered after the first ring and I could not contain my emotions.

"Not good, Scott. Why do some people not care?"

"What is going on?" Scott questioned with great concern.

"Dad is not well; you better come."

"Okay, Melissa and I will drive up in a couple hours. How are you?"

"Exhausted. Nurse last night was so horrible. Always would have to get him to give dad his meds and would be at his workstation on the computer and was not affected when I told him dad was suffering."

"I would have done something more than just talking to him," Scott was livid.

"Trust me I wanted to, but dad would be upset if something happened. You know him and not wanting to make waves."

"Kay, going to sort things out here and hit the road soon. Call me on my cell and keep me posted."

"Will do. Careful driving."

I hung up and drove to my mom's where I had a shower and lunch. After lunch, I called my cousin Paul who lived nearby and I would head over to his place to have a beverage and talk.

Paul was the oldest of my aunt's three sons and his two brothers were closer to me and my brother's age. Because of the age gap, dad and Paul had a greater bond and Paul would be included in events with dad and his brothers when they would visit.

"What would you like?" Paul asked.

"Ginger ale would be fine, thanks," I replied.

We sat outside on Paul's patio as it was such a sunny, beautiful day. We didn't say much.

"Dad is not good, Paul, afraid not much longer. Scott and Melissa are driving up."

"Sucks," Paul replied with anguish.

I took my first sip of ginger ale when my phone received a text, was my cousin Ruth who was staying with dad. The text read, "Greg, where are you?"

I replied that I was at my cousin Paul's, resting and visiting. Ruth responded with "You better come."

I placed my beverage down and told Paul I had to go and that this did not sound good. I drove as fast as I could and was conflicted. Was this bad dad's life was coming to an end? He suffered so much for so long and could not get better but only worse.

I parked my car and ran as fast as I could, becoming emotional as I ran. The hallway towards dad's room seemed never-ending. As I turned the corner, Ruth stood outside dad's room, shaking her head to tell me dad was gone. I bent over and placed my hands on my knees and let out some loud groans which caused staff to look. I tried to control my breathing but was having great difficulty which resulted in more groans.

I finally did control my breathing, standing up and walking in to dad's room where he lay on his back covered to his chest. His face did not have an oxygen mask on and the machines around him were silent. I hugged him and held him, kissing his cheek and beginning to cry again.

After hugging Cathy and Ruth, Ruth described what had happened.

"When the nurse injected his first increase dosage of medication, I noticed his breathing became shallower and he slowly stopped, he did not suffer."

I was so thrilled he did not suffer and went peacefully. Dad fought through that last night even with that nurse's care provided to him, I was so proud of my father.

I went out in the hallway and called my brother. After the fourth ring, which did not surprise me as Scott knew the news I was about to deliver, he answered.

"Hey."

"He is gone," I said, beginning to cry.

"Okay we are about three hours away, "Scott replied, becoming emotional as I heard my sister Melissa crying in the background.

"Come directly to the hospital and you can see dad," I said.

Dad passing in the early afternoon and the undertaker unable to arrive quickly, we were allowed to let dad remain in his room till Scott and Melissa arrived. This would allow them to see and grieve dad alone as he would next be seen at his viewing at the funeral home in four days.

As Cathy, Ruth and I waited, I went and grabbed a blanket and covered dad. I noticed he was starting to change just in the short time since he passed.

Dad fought so hard and I am so proud I can tell people he gave cancer a 15-round fight. Maybe dad should have received the increase in medication long ago but he wanted to fight and this was dad's decision to make even though the fight was horrible to watch. I also was proud but saddened he had to fight with some who provided care to him, his nurse that last night.

I did not work in end-of-life care but saw such amazing nurses in my work and life experience who, by just asking how we were as we watched our loved one struggle, made you feel you were not alone.

Scott and Melissa arrived and walked into the room, visibly upset. Scott approached dad and pulled the blanket back, kissing him on the forehead. When he did, I became emotional not only from my brother's loving gesture but also at how shocking dad looked. I could not recognize him as just in the few hours his physical appearance had changed dramatically and was a memory I have to erase. After Melissa had her moment with dad, we said good bye to Cathy and Ruth who would wait for the undertaker.

Before the three us left, I did get the nurse's full name as well as his manager's, Dr. Hook, from his fellow nurses who tended to dad with care and compassion his final morning and administered his last medication. They did not hesitate with the information, seeming almost excited to give it to me.

Looking back, I wish I would have gone further reporting the care Robert gave to the College of Nurses. This college was there to protect the public, us, from nurses like Robert.

As we left, we did not see the nurse. I was disappointed but glad as having my brother with me and who has dad's temper, things would have gotten ugly. The Soo is not a big place and I will see him at some point. I can hopefully stop him from treating others this way, not from physically hurting him which I wanted to do but with the information I had gathered.

CHAPTER SEVENTEEN

Good with the Bad

Dear Dr. Hook:

My name is Greg Noack and my father, Lennox Hiram Issac Noack, was a patient numerous times at your Hospital due to complications from lung cancer and Chronic Obstructive Pulmonary Disorder (COPD). His last stay was for well over two weeks on floor 4 East.

My dad always told me to talk about the good with the bad and I am going to do this regarding my experiences at your Hospital from August 28th - August 31st.

When I arrived to see my father on Wednesday afternoon, August 28th, my heart broke as this man who was once full of life and laughter now lay supine in a hospital bed with an oxygen mask on as well as nose prongs to keep him breathing. I told my father he could go and leave us but he stated he wasn't going anywhere. I am so proud of his fight but was saddened as I knew my father was suffering and fighting a battle he could not win. He was fighting for those he loved.

I decided to spend that night with my dad to give my stepmother Cathy a break as she would spend every hour of the day if she could with dad but I was concerned about her and caregiver burden.

So, I spent Wednesday night with dad and was so impressed by his night nurse Shenise. She would come in every hour and check on dad and if an injection of medicine was needed, she would talk to dad and let him know what was going on.

My father had a tendency to pull his oxygen mask off and become agitated, sensing it was preventing him from breathing; stressing even greater the importance to check in on my father, along with his inability to use the call bell to get help. I did not sleep well and when I did dose off would be woken by Shenise checking on dad, which I did not mind as I was worried if I had fallen asleep, dad would have pulled that oxygen mask off. I feared my father suffocating and not dying peacefully.

Over the next 36 hours, my dad's condition deteriorated and an increase of medication that helped ease the pain and his agitation was implemented. During the time I spent over those 36 hours, I was impressed by the care my dad received. The nurses were empathetic and caring with each new nurse I saw treating dad in this manner (Thomas and Shenise).

This all changed on Friday evening, as Robert was my dad's nurse. He was different from the 'Good' from his initial interaction with dad. My stepmother Cathy and I sensed it was going to be a long night as when Robert came in to see dad to begin his shift, he never introduced himself to us or dad and actually was whistling a song as he was tending to my father.

Cathy who is so thoughtful tried to open up discussion with Robert and create friendly banter but was met with little interest and a response of exasperation: "Working tonight and the weekend, which is fun."

From the whistling and the short response to Cathy, I wondered if Robert was in the right profession, tending to the needs of patients and their families experiencing what we were. There was no compassion or empathy present.

My father never wanted any of us to 'rock the boat' in regard to his care but I knew this would be difficult not to do with Robert.

I stayed with my dad that last night and Cathy unwillingly left but made a point to tell Robert to check in on dad as I may fall asleep and we were both very concerned with dad's tendency of pulling his oxygen mask off.

This is where a chart review/investigation may be in order as I was confused with what medication my father was to receive. Dad's agitation was increasing as well as his pain so I was under the impression he would receive morphine every hour.

8:15pm: Robert gave my dad a morphine injection so I would wait till 9:15 to see if he would receive one. 9:15 came along and I working in health care for over 12 years gave Robert 15 minutes extra, understanding how a nurse's caseload can be heavy.

9:30pm: I used the call bell and Robert finally came. He gave my father his injection and left the room. What bothered me was he never talked to my dad and I even said thank you as to not 'rock the boat' as dad would want and I did not receive 'you're welcome or no problem'. Robert just sanitized his hands and left the room.

I was getting tired so I decided to try to get some sleep but really could not because I was concerned. I was so worried dad would take that oxygen mask off and suffocate. But I also knew if dad received that injection every hour, he may not come to that point. I had my brother call my cell phone at 11:00 so I would be awake just in case.

11:00pm: An hour and a half had gone by, with Robert not checking in. I used the call bell and Robert finally came. I said it was time for dad's morphine and Robert said dad is resting and that it is not necessary. Being ignorant of morphine, I did not say anything but was perplexed a bit. Looking back, I wish I inquired more.

11:05pm to 3:00am: I slipped in and out of consciousness and really can't give a definite answer of the care my father received. I would wake up on Wednesday night when dad's nurse, Shenise, came in but did not this night.

3:05am: My father yelled and I popped up, he took his oxygen mask off and was agitated. I held his mask on and used the call bell for Robert. He came in and gave dad his injection of morphine. He stated he gave him one at 1:30 and I thought to myself *'the math does not work'*, that is two and half hours from 11:00 when he did not receive his shot. A possible four hours without something that may have made my dad comfortable if Robert had not come like he said at 1:30. I am ignorant of morphine but do question if given every hour, would my dad have become agitated like this and suffer?

3:00am-7:00am: Will always be the hardest four hours of my life. I pulled a chair up beside dad and held his hand and talked to him as dad would let out intermittent groans. I also would make sure dad was checked in on and given what was needed to make him comfortable.

4:00am: An hour had passed since my father's last injection and check in. I used the call bell and Robert arrived. He gave dad his injection and I 'rocked the boat' even though my father could hear. Robert said he had come in to check dad and that he was asleep and I confronted him, stating, "You did not as I was wide awake holding my dad's hand as he groaned." Robert did not respond, gave dad his injection and left the room.

4:30am: My dad's breathing was becoming very labored so I went to Robert who was sitting at workstation on the computer eating a snack and asked if my dad could have Ventolin, a medicine that temporarily opens up my father's airway so he could breathe easier and Robert responded with 'Really no point'. I would later find out dad could have had this, which really made me question Robert's work ethic and if he followed the standards of the College of Nurses. Sitting at the computer eating chips was more important than my father being comfortable.

5:00am: Robert entered the room without my calling and gave dad his injection. He then left and I did not see him again.

6:55am: I stepped out of my father's room and Robert was at the elevator going home. I was confused by even this as I work in a Rehab hospital in Toronto and at shift change, the nurses collaborated with one another and talked face-to-face about their patients and what had been occurring with their care before leaving.

After Robert had left, I was exhausted and confused by the night's events as I angrily vented to Thomas who was beginning his shift. I would like to apologize to him for doing this and hope this can be passed on.

I composed myself and after the 'Bad' was greeted with the 'Good'. Nurses Carolina and Gloria cared for my father in his final hours and were so amazing. So much so Cathy and I mention them in my father's obituary. I sensed their pain from my father's suffering, along with ours.

I noticed they did things that made dad comfortable, something Robert did not do. They put a port in dad's side for him to receive his morphine. Robert kept on pricking my father's belly over and over when maybe he could have avoided this by doing the same. Carolina and Gloria also talked to my dad with such kindness and compassion, something my father did not receive from Robert.

1:10pm: My father died peacefully at approximately this time on August 31st, and I am so grateful to the nurses that were with him and us at that time.

My father would want me to write this letter as he would not want another patient to experience the care he received that night and I am proud as well as sad in writing this. What will haunt me is what if I wasn't there advocating for my dad, I know Robert would not have checked in and made my dad comfortable and my father would have removed that oxygen mask, suffocating and not pass peacefully.

An empathetic colleague and esteemed doctor who I work with said I have to write this and now let it go for dad's sake or it will eat at me. I have gotten it out and will not lie and say I won't still have moments regarding my father's last night, and this is the impact the care Robert provided to my father has had on me and my family. I do take solace in the fact that I was there for my father and he received a very deserving peaceful end.

In summary, I request the following:

1) A full review of the care given to my father, particularly Friday night.
2) Did this follow your Hospital policies, procedures, and best practice?
3) If something can be learned regarding my father's care, can this provide education to prevent future incidents?
4) An apology to Thomas for my heated feedback.

This letter was written for my father, my stepmother Cathy, my cousin Ruthie, the advocating family and those who do not have someone to watch over them.

Love you dad and I 'rocked the boat' for a good reason.
Sincerely, Greg Noack (Lil' LEN)

LIL' Fighter

Dad's funeral would be held on a Tuesday, with a visitation Monday evening. The visitation was for three hours, and we stood in line greeting people as they came to pay their respects. Dad had an open casket and the funeral home did an amazing job on how he looked compared to when I saw him when he passed and how he looked just a few hours later.

We all stood in line, forming a half circle with dad's open casket at the midpoint. Cathy and I, my brother and sisters stood at the beginning of the line followed by my dad's brothers and sisters, a majority who came from Pembroke, where my dad was born. It was great to see them and reminisce about dad.

The home was nice and before you came to the room where my father was lying, there was an area with pictures of dad and a slide show being played continuously on a large screen with photos of him as a teenager to before he became ill. The viewing was from 6 to 9, 3 hours and was very draining. 300 people came showing dad's popularity and that he touched many peoples' lives.

The viewing was emotional throughout but more so when Carmen came through. I told her how moved I was by her coming and also mentioned her stepdaughter Irene being as gentle with dad as his nurse just five days earlier. My principal from high school and his wife came, as his son was my best friend in high school and could not be there. Mr. Mando was not only my principal and best friend's father but a loving influence when I was growing up.

The visitation was like a time warp bringing back so many memories of my life with dad. In the moment, you don't realize how life is fleeting and goes by in an instant and you should cherish those moments.

The next day was dad's funeral which would be held at the chapel room attached to the funeral home. I would talk last after my brother, two sisters, and stepbrother, Kevin. Kevin's daughter Carissa would end the ceremony singing Amazing Grace. I was adamant she end the ceremony because, with her voice, singing that song at the beginning would make me an emotional wreck; was going to be anyway.

I was so impressed by my siblings and I know dad would be. I begin my talk, stating this and then began my eulogy.

"What did my dad teach me? He taught me how to fight and give 100%.

I think back to about 13 years ago, when I was in Pembroke, his home town, and when I went to where he grew up.

It was a small three-bedroom home with no electricity and no access to roads. It amazed me that he and 10 others lived under this one roof and they lived off the land. As my Uncle Dennis stated, when the chicken stopped laying eggs, it was in the pot for dinner. Seeing this, I realized where he and his brothers and sisters, us Noacks, established that fighting spirit.

Dad always showed me the importance of family as he adored when with, or talking about, his brothers Dennis, Howard, Clarence, and sisters, Mona, Euena, Goldie and Myrtle.

Dad also showed me how to give 100% in a lot of areas of life from work to family. With work, dad went off and managed department stores in Toronto, what courage from an Ottawa Valley boy and after, own and run his own restaurant. Dad's last job was at the Casino, from dealer to cash supervisor to ending at the Coat Check, which he loved because he could socialize. When it came to work, dad always told me to be on time, 'be committed to what you do and dress the part'.

This showed even recently as this past November when he began his fight with cancer and when I came up to see him when he was in ICU, the first thing he said to me was "Was work okay with this?"

With children, Dad loved his kids and when I was little always wanted to give us: me, Scott, Kim and Melissa the best, which looking back sadly I think consumed dad when we were smaller as not having much himself he wanted to give us it all.

He ended up giving us it all as we got older, and was so thrilled when the family expanded, as Kim married Bob and blessed us with Hanna; Scott married Amy and blessed us with Stella, and Melissa married Dan and blessed us with Lyla. Dad would always light up and be so proud of his grandchildren.

My dad also blessed us with more family as he met and married Cathy, Ma #2 as I like to call her. With Cathy, dad gained another son, Kevin and three more girls, Elaine, Tara and Christine. And from them Val, who with Kevin gave my dad Courtney and Carissa (George as I like to call her, a nickname I took from dad). Al, who with Christine gave us Ryan and Max, and Sean and Tara, who gave us Chaffon. Dad loved all the little ones as he would tell me stories, some repeated, and I received so much joy from them.

Now the difficult part, where dad really showed me how to fight and give 100%. And here is where he would like me to fight through this and expand on certain people and things.

November 13th, 2012 a day which I found out my father would take on another fight, this with lung cancer. He fought so courageously for nine months.

He would want to thank Cathy, and I would like to thank her as well, for being with Dad and giving so much to him, not just with this fight but for the past 22 years, as Dad would tell me stories about you, some repeated, and be so proud and in love. Thank you Ma #2. You are forever this to me and this will never change, I love you. And the way you were with Dad at the end showed me what true unconditional love is.

He would like me to give thanks to Kevin, Val, Elaine, Courtney, Carissa and Eric, and I will as well because you were here for dad during his final fight and you represented those of us who couldn't, giving our love to him through yourselves.

Dad would thank his niece Ruthie and her husband Jack. Dad viewed you as a daughter Ruthie, and I am so thrilled you introduced him to your church and Reverend John, as I believe Dad found peace with God and is looking down on us, and I will see him again.

I will end with something Dad mentioned to Cathy. The reason my Dad had to fight was because of smoking, and if I did not mention Dad's habit for 50 years, something I am so proud he quit over five years ago, he would feel there would not be a reason for the fight he gave: to show us the damage, hurt, and pain smoking can do.

Smoking took my Dad away, I was very blessed to have him for over

41 years but wish I could have him for more. I have people here today who I love dearly, who do smoke and I pray you learn what this addiction does from my father, the fighter and giver of 100%.

Love you, Dad! And my final words to you were that you will continue to live through me and I won't let you down. I will forever be Lil' Len.

Let it go

When I returned to work, I was in a daze. I was hypersensitive before towards how my colleagues treated patients but now this was even more magnified seeing it through the eyes of a caregiver with my father.

The nine months after dad's diagnosis aged me and my fatigue which is my biggest deficit would overwhelm me at times. The first week was very difficult as I would receive sympathy from my colleagues and the retelling of dad's last night drove me to tears every time.

An amazing doctor and close friend of mine who I worked alongside of in research warned me not to be enveloped by dad's treatment at the end.

So, I wrote a letter three days after my return to work to the manager of the floor that my father was on and specifically detailed our last night and the interactions we had with dad's nurse. Like writing ***My Invisible Disability*** and now my second book the letter was cathartic and allowed me to get what was bothering me out. Hopefully then I could follow my colleague's advice of not dwelling on this memory of dad, something he would not want me to do. 'The good with bad' titled letter was the hardest thing I have written and my proudest piece of work.

Almost a week had gone by when I received an email back from the manager. The response was what I expected, having worked in healthcare over the years, with no one wanting to do the work to solve the issues. I was familiar with manager speak and the diplomacy involved in defending your staff even when they were undoubtedly in the wrong.

The manager did do a chart review and stated it was to Robert's discretion and along with his assessment as to when to give my father morphine. He also stated Robert administered the morphine while I slept. This annoyed me as the nurse on the previous time I spent the evening with dad was like clockwork, every hour, and comforting my father as she administered the morphine. I knew every hour because I awoke every time, she came in. Odd I did not wake when Robert came in.

To me, the response was a way to defend Robert's laziness and lack of empathy. The manager did not mention in his email Robert not wanting to pull away from his computer and early morning snack to give my father medication that would allow him to breathe easier and decrease his suffering when I asked him to. I was not at all satisfied with this and expressed so in my reply back.

"Good morning Mr. Hook, I appreciate the letter and response. I am not totally satisfied with the outcome and for the sake of others; I hope the nurse in question does not deal with dying patients and their loved ones in the future." Regards, Greg.

Unlike my original email I received a reply within the hour.

"Hi, Greg. I realize my response is vague with regard to the action taken with Robert and this doesn't sit well with you. I'm very limited in what I'm able to disclose due to confidentiality but I do want to assure you that the issues were addressed. Thank you."

My letter to management was good to send and get things off my chest. That was the only good thing to come of it as my friend who works at the hospital stated Robert was still working in the same way. His colleagues would voice their complaints but the care he provided continued unabated.

CHAPTER EIGHTEEN

Players

I had a meeting with my manager. He was the fourth manager I worked under. His position was viewed as a stepping stone to other higher executive positions, thus the turnover. The four all had different approaches and backgrounds through their own work experience and education.

I respected my newest manager the most as he was educated on the management of people and came from another hospital, meaning he was not friends with those he managed.

The managers before were internal, hired from within, using the position as a rung on the ladder to climb towards bigger things. I was not fond of this especially in the health care industry. I realized like any other industry, along with the time you put in, who you knew and what you said can be beneficial in regard to promotion. Sometimes words were put before actions.

I also understood people had to grow in their profession and promotion is required as I witnessed some who may have stayed too long in their role. This led to burnout or even the loss of someone valuable to the field.

By being internal and promoted from within, managers were sometimes reluctant to reprimand poor performance and may have had greater concern about being liked, ignoring the issues of those they worked alongside of prior to being a manager. I found it odd that one of my previous managers was friends with a majority of his staff on social media platforms.

I would tell these managers some of my colleagues' performance issues and nothing would come of it. The culture of friendship or tolerance started at the top and would trickle down, resulting in poor patient care. The stream flows downward and if pollution is at the top, this makes everything polluted along the way. I worked hard and was rewarded with witnessing the gains of persons with a brain injury who I rehabilitated. I did not want to climb the ladder and focused on this. I did not use optics, saying and doing things to impress, and took my job seriously. I wanted to be judged by the care I provided, my actions. I questioned why some of my colleagues may have not taken their job seriously like I did.

Upon admission to the rehab hospital, a patient was assigned a team of professionals; a primary nurse, OT, PT, SLP, SW, Rehab Therapist and if needed Behavior Therapist and depending on who, if they were part of my team in 1996, I would have never had the recovery and outcome I had.

Harsh words but to me true. One member of the team could prevent a patient from regaining a better quality of life and not being discharged home to their loved ones. Sadly, I witnessed substandard care by someone from each profession, meaning a patient had a very remote chance but still a chance of having all five members of their team providing care that affected their rehab outcome.

I am grateful for the care I received in my rehabilitation from brain injury and extremely grateful for being Canadian due to the government covering the cost of my rehabilitation. Down south in the US, I cannot imagine the cost of close to a year of rehabilitation. I know my family would have had to mortgage their future for me to have another chance at one.

A positive I did see in the US business model of health care was you needed to be the best to attract patients and poor performance was not tolerated or accepted. I found in Canada from my involvement with hospitals be it as a patient, clinician, and family member that the "It is free so don't complain" sentiment created complacency. This created health care professionals who saw the dollar sign over the patient and were more willing to climb the ladder to receive greater dollars.

Several colleagues I started with ten plus years ago moved on to other positions and did not work on the front line anymore. A majority deserved to move up but the younger inexperienced replacements did not have their work ethic and this difference annoyed me.

Viewing our jobs like any other and as a stepping stone for other positions irked me as we were dealing with vulnerable people who needed us at our best for another chance at an acceptable quality of life. This attitude along with the protection of a union for some made the fear of dismissal nonexistent and in fact joked about.

I was part of the union as an occupational therapist assistant and the fees I paid I questioned as I know sometimes the union would go to 'bat' for someone who may have used the power of the union to protect their poor performance.

"You're late again."

"Go tell the manager. What is he going to do?"

A confident response given from a therapist in a conversation I overheard amongst colleagues. I am very fortunate this therapist was not mine when I went through rehabilitation.

This was the third sit down with my newest manager. Our previous two meetings dealt with how I was coping with my father's passing. My manager sensed my preoccupation with the loss of dad. I struggled with this for a year when my manager suggested I speak to a counsellor, a service provided by the hospital to its employees.

I accepted and after six sessions that focused on going through the grieving process, I was finally at peace. This process allowed me to let go of other losses that I never thought of. The biggest being the loss of my former self that died on that bridge in Victoria, BC eighteen years earlier.

In the first year after my brain injury, all I concentrated on was getting better and restoring my life to its fullest potential. I had an amazing support system, my mother being the greatest, and was blessed with a unique, almost spontaneous, and miraculous recovery from brain injury. In fact, I feel it was meant to be and God's plan with the path my life had taken.

I was left with deficits, fatigue being my biggest and struggle with the thoughts that old, pre brain injury Greg may have excelled in my first career path of business/human resources and met the expectations of having a wife and children, having ample energy to pursue and achieve such expectations. I will never know.

Grieving the loss of my father allowed me to grieve the potential of old Greg and put those thoughts to rest, dad's last gift to me. A gift I wanted to share with other persons with a brain injury.

I rehabilitated persons with a brain injury in their first couple months after injury and grieving their former self was farthest from their mind. But what about six months down the road to recovery when the reality of their changed self sets in and they do not know how to mourn the person they were before brain injury?

I wanted to expand on this with my manager and, working in research the past three years, I look forward to dissecting grief in persons with a brain injury. This would be discussed in another meeting; this one was going to be about my work environment, more importantly some of those working in it.

I approached his open door, a policy he had from his first day, meaning if something was on your mind or any issues that were concerning, you could discuss with him. I grabbed us each a coffee, guess I played 'the game' too, but I didn't purchase his coffee to get ahead, but as a token of appreciation for listening to what I had to say and in the hope that we could make a change. Hopefully he was tired of the games being played.

Insanity

"Afternoon Walt."

Walter Walker was two years into his job as my manager. I got the okay to call him Walt when I first met him. I did this when I first met patients as well. I would call them Mr. or Mrs. and once given their permission would call them by their first names. This was a simple and effective way to build rapport which showed the patient respect.

I would hear colleagues of mine say a patient's first name on their initial interaction without getting permission and one colleague would call them kids, even though they themselves were quite younger. I found both objectionable.

"Thanks for the coffee. How are you, Greg?" Walt asked.

Walt always asked me this first and was in regard to the counselling I received grieving dad. The sessions ended months ago but he wanted to make sure I was still coping.

"Things are good. Thanks again for helping me with the loss of dad. Want to chat with you about what is happening on the floor. Hate being a snitch, but feel patient care is being affected."

"You are not being a snitch. I am not a micro manager and do not have the time to be in all places, so you telling me keeps me aware of what is happening on the floor and with our patients."

"Kay. A couple of colleagues seem to come in late quite a bit for years now and by doing so patients are not getting proper ADL (activities of daily life) practice."

This flustered me as a patient not being able to practice their shower and dressing routine due to someone not being on time could result in that patient not going home. I would cover for my colleagues because of this probability but was starting to burnout and becoming more frustrated, frustrated at the referring therapists as well. Why didn't they give them feedback, trying to solve the problem? If I was five minutes late, they were quick to give me feedback.

"I know who you are talking about. This is a chronic issue. This tardiness has been going on for so long that it is accepted and tolerated. I am looking into the matter."

I had heard that Walt waited in our office and caught one of the late arrivers previously and that it was being closely monitored.

My first career path in human resources I learned how difficult it was to terminate an employee. The process of termination was long and tedious and the onus fell on the manager to build a case for dismissal.

I also was educated by a chat I had with a colleague who was very high up and ran another hospital in regard to managing such situations. This colleague questioned if our managers looked into what was causing the lateness and could these peoples' schedules be changed to meet their needs and more importantly not interfere with the care we provided?

I knew you had to be careful as well as managers over the years would state "Greg, we can't confront workers who may need help and possibly stigmatize them."

This response perplexed me as if I struggled with not being on time from issues that could be alleviated with help I would want that help. Also, my struggles should not be to the detriment of those in need of help. Ignoring my problem would result in collateral damage, patients not getting care.

This was bothersome to me. I have family who work in the auto industry and if someone was late and it affected production, they would not last long. Being late for putting cars together should not be equivalent or of greater importance than putting people lives back together.

"There is talk that you are looking into it. Just don't get it. If I knew my manager was keeping a close eye on me, I would make it a priority to be on time and even early," I said.

"I know. For years, getting away with such behavior gives this person a sense of invincibility," Walt replied.

"Still why test it? Quick question, you don't have to answer, but how hard is it to get rid of someone?"

I knew the answer but asked anyway. I could see the irritation on Walt's face before he responded.

"Very difficult, it is a lot of work to justify the reason for termination," Walt replied.

"There is the problem, just have troubles grasping all of this," I responded.

"Your expectations for your job and how you work is high, Greg. When people don't meet them, you get angry and you can't let this eat at you or you will become miserable," Walt advised me.

"I know, but working in an environment that allows minimum expectations from my profession bothers me. And I feel I am the only one it bugs. Sad thing is if my performance is off, say late a few minutes, the referring therapists are quick to give me feedback. Why not them?" I asked.

"This drives me nuts, Greg, but you're expected to be on point because you have been a reliable, hard worker from day one. The therapists can count on you and rely on you. If you were like the chronic late person, they would shrug it off and expect it."

What he stated made sense. Referring therapists, I am sure, complained to previous managers about this person and this issue but since nothing happened, it became useless to try to correct and became easier to ignore. This performance was now expected of that person and accepted. They were normalizing this behavior.

"And your job is so large, Walt, you don't have time to babysit. Would be great if you did not have so much on your plate and could be out there on the floor."

"I know, Greg."

When Walt first started, he met with each professional group and stated his expectations of us, one being on time for starting and finishing your scheduled shift. Something he reiterated at staff meetings over his two years and at our last meeting, he became very blunt and direct regarding this expectation.

In the month after his stern reminder, the usual suspects would still come and go as they pleased. They knew Walt had larger concerns to tend to than observe our comings and goings. Walt gave us great autonomy and some were taking advantage of this.

What bothered both of us was this culture was not putting patients first and was affecting their care. And even a greater concern was that others, more than I thought, had the same mindset as the usual suspects making this culture acceptable.

Walt sent all of us a survey electronically with four choices and we had to rank what we felt was most important in our working environment. I ranked interprofessional collaboration and team building number one and two. These two items, to me, if focused on, would lead to optimum patient care.

I was in the minority as the most popular choices were accommodating flexibility of employees' schedules and staff recognition. I was embarrassed by this. My colleagues wanted even more autonomy along with recognition of a job well done. We thought of ourselves first and not the patients we rehabilitated. They did not grasp the fact that, if not for the patients suffering a traumatic brain injury, they would not have their jobs.

After discussing both our frustrations in greater detail, more me than Walt, I ended by thanking him for listening and said I hope to not be the only one who reported these issues. He repeated to me not to feel this way and to keep voicing my concerns to him and that his door was always open.

As I left and walked down the hallway, I did not feel alone. Maybe a change could occur, but I am not stupid. Patients were getting free care and should be happy with whatever they received. My coffees with Walt occurred less over time.

Break

I was meeting with Walt for the first time in six months. Tried to cool it on my frequency of meeting with him as I did not want to come across as disgruntled and what I would say to him then would have less impact. Walt is a great manager with too much to deal with already and I did not want to add to this.

I loved my job and wanted to have another 20 years, but my aggravation for parts of my job were continuing to grow. I felt some of my colleagues were more eager to please one another than the patients we rehabilitated. I may have been guilty of this to a degree as well.

How Walt viewed me was crucial due to him being my manager but most important to me was how the patients viewed me and the job I did. I did not work to impress the therapists whose treatment programs I carried out. I was not their servant but their patients'.

The hierarchy found in most workplaces was rampant at my job. Walt expressed to us his aggravation with this and wanted from doctors to house keepers treated equally. I worked with some who fed the hierarchy, ignoring patient care to run errands for the people they perceived above them. What was sad is the therapists whose patients were ignored said nothing due to the colleague would drop what they were doing to serve them.

My wonderful friend and doctor who I worked alongside of in research said it best, "Greg, we work with personalities, not professionals."

I could not agree more with her statement. I am a very rigid, partial to my injury to the frontal lobe of my brain, and also am hypersensitive to the cause, having gone through what those who I rehabilitated did. I got annoyed if others did not meet my expectations. Being this way, I became a glutton for more work and by doing more work covered for the poor performance of others. I was told to let things be and not interject and things would come to light. I would but after the light was shining like a beacon and nothing would be done to solve the problem, I would go back to covering for others. What was sad is the job would get done and that was all that mattered to those who ran the hospital.

"Hi, Walt."

I entered his office with a coffee for each of us. I set our coffees down on the table in his office that we would sit at and then shut the door.

"How are things going?" Walt asked.

"Broken record. Find sadly a high number of my colleagues are more focused on impressing one another and their own professional goals than those of their patients. And the others things I have brought to your attention before keep recurring."

My colleagues continuing to come and go as they pleased, cutting therapy sessions short by being late or ending early. Some did not even show for their scheduled treatment sessions. I was always perplexed that if we could not manage punctuality, how could you tackle the deeper performance issues?

The year I spent in the Soo working in long term care, the facility had a swipe card system, basically a punch clock. Your ID badge had a bar code on it which you swiped in a machine when you entered and left. If someone was late, a message would be sent electronically to the manager's computer and if this person's tardiness continued, warnings were given and if late after that, termination. The swipe card system also monitored when staff left and if the time leaving was past their scheduled shift, the reason for this was looked into as well.

Some reasons for going beyond your shift could be theft or productivity. When I worked in LTC, I heard someone was swiping after their scheduled shift was over and the matter was looked into. Turned out this staff was stealing from the residents.

Regarding productivity, I know Walt had 12-hour shifts and if others above him, his boss, knew of the many extra hours he put in maybe help would be given resulting in less burnout and turnover in the managerial position. I brought the swipe card idea to Walt and others before him and nothing came of it.

"I don't understand, Greg. You voice your concerns to me and it is appreciated and I am aware of it myself but if it is just you and not a collective that state this problem, it is very hard for me to move forward on the issue."

Made sense, would be my word against their word which is not enough evidence. No one wanted to be the bad guy and the culture of friendship really played the part in this. Walt and I conversed for a couple hours and felt good to know he agreed with me in a majority of my views about the environment we both worked in.

He was aware of the younger professionals and their sense of entitlement caused in part by the hierarchy that existed. The title after your name seemed to give you the ability to work less on the front line and focus on what could make your work title more prestigious.

"Greg, as we discussed previously, you and I have greater expectations in regard to how someone performs. Others don't meet these expectations but rather view their job as meeting their obligations. If they meet these, they feel they have done their duty. As a manager, I really have difficulty reprimanding someone if they meet the obligations of their job but fail to meet expectations."

Walt opened my eyes with what he said. This also was sad as how could we inspire others to be better and meet expectations instead of just obligations.

My colleague, who is late all the time and sits around doing nothing or does the minimal of what is expected, does show up and meets that obligation and nothing more. That I am the only one it seems to bother will always frustrate me.

"Question for you, Walt. How many people are just here to meet the obligations of their job and not bother with the higher expectations you and I have?"

I wanted to say roughly 40 percent. I was surprised by Walt's response, "More like 65 percent."

"That high?" I questioned.

"Yes, sadly. Times are changing, Greg. The younger generation is focused on more than frontline work and remaining there. They want to go beyond their clinical work and seek other opportunities. They meet their obligations and nothing more so they can have time to pursue other avenues. If they met our high expectations, there would be little time for pursuing other avenues."

He was correct. And I do not fault my colleagues for this. What bothered me, and I am sure Walt, is they put their career aspirations first over patient care. If it was the other way around, I would not be questioning their performance.

"Well, Walt, thanks for your time and making me see things differently. It helps."

"No problem. Door is always open."

Sadly, it would not be open anymore. Walt would announce his sudden resignation two months later to all of our shock. He was moving back home and getting out of health care. He was the best manager I had ever worked with and how he viewed where we worked was very similar to mine. The 65 percent got to him and if I managed this percentage with such attitudes and could not change them, I would have lasted only four months, not four years.

Walt had met more than his obligations and by doing so may have burnt himself out. He will be missed.

CHAPTER NINETEEN

Exemplary

"Why didn't you sue the doctor who did this to you?" I asked Bob.

I was three months post my brain injury and starting my second month of outpatient rehabilitation. I was still lost in finding my way spiritually. I questioned my mortality and why I was spared while others were less fortunate.

"Well, Greg, the doctor made a mistake and his mistakes are more profound, but I am sure he is an amazing doctor and surgeon."

I was flabbergasted by Bob's response but was not surprised. He was such a positive and inspirational human being. I would later find out that the surgeon who tended to me was the one who worked on Bob. Bob's story was an example for me to follow, over 20 years later.

I did find God and was born again a year after my injury but was having difficulty forgiving my colleagues and their poor performance.

Giving feedback was extremely difficult for me. This involved confrontation which I feared and my assault reinforced this. My history also gave the person I gave feedback to an excuse.

"Greg is being too sensitive and overreacting," I would hear.

My mother said it best in regard to my situation, "Greg, it is sad but your coworkers will judge what you are saying by your history and not by its merit."

Mom was correct but this irritated me. So, if I didn't have a brain injury, would the person be more accepting of my feedback?

I recall the first time I shared my story with the patients I rehabilitated. Several of my colleagues were in the audience and one in particular made sure I was aware of my brain injury and the deficits brought on by it.

"So, Greg, do you find you are more open and say things that maybe you should not than before your injury?" my colleague asked.

I was thrown off by her question and stammered with my response.

"Not too much I think, hard to gauge as I really can't remember how I was before my injury."

"It seems you do," she replied.

I was surprised she did not let my response go and seemed to me she was attempting to make a point. I replied to her curt response.

"Well maybe I am. Being honest and open makes me a great clinician and a trait my brain injury brought out of me, I view it as a blessing."

The patients in the audience liked my answer and that is what mattered to me, even though my colleague shrugged it off as to imply I was wrong.

This interaction made me view her differently. How did she interact with her patients that she treated? Was it her goal to hammer home a patient's deficits or to work on these deficits and help her patients move past them?

Over the years, a few patients would share their displeasure with me in how therapists were out to prove their brain injury affected them and how they were different from someone without one. I understood the importance of building insight for the patients and building awareness of their deficits, preparing them for the changes brought on by their brain injury physically and mentally. Then providing compensatory strategies to help them function close to who they were pre brain injury and most importantly live safely, preventing another brain injury.

Sadly, some would not gain this insight and try to live the life they once had. My swimming friend Vincent in Victoria was this way and I would have been this way as well. Taking risks to be who you once were is a gamble I would take and this gamble can be perceived as having lack of insight. I was extremely fortunate gaining insight and perspective from my brain injury but, to me, these were also a deficit.

My employment in rehabilitation of those who suffered a similar fate as me highlighted this as I wanted all to have an outcome like mine. If the people who I worked alongside prevented patients achieving this and in turn upset them and their family, it personally affected me.

I am guilty of building patients up too much my one colleague stated and maybe I did. I preferred to be this way than breaking them down even more in their most vulnerable state. How I worked followed the "Don't kick a person when they are down" adage. I also have to remember what Bob did, and put things in a better perspective. He forgave someone who took away his ability to walk and in doing so that same person helped me.

My colleagues did amazing work but sometimes would falter and let some patients down. None of us are perfect and I have to remind myself to put things in perspective. In my now 20 years of work in rehabilitation, no one made a mistake causing someone to lose their ability to walk, maybe they just prevented them in regaining the ability to do so.

Surprises

"Wish we had a chair," my colleague stated.

I had a confused look on my face and asked, "What do you mean?"

"Someone who is in a wheelchair who would share their story about brain injury to the patients we have on the floor. I have one recently discharged patient who is ambulatory and looks normal who will be presenting, would be nice to have someone with physical impairment to show the varying outcomes of brain injury."

I was thrown off by the initial question, seemed cold and ignoring of the person who is in that chair.

"I may have someone. I will let you know," I said.

"Awesome, Greg. Keep me posted."

I had reconnected with Peter, a person I rehabilitated 10 years earlier. The hospital has an excellent volunteer program and he had become one. He would go room to room in his power wheelchair and share his plight with patients individually.

We would talk and reminisce about when we first met, him a patient and me a therapy assistant. We chuckled at the morning showers I assisted him with and how I worked on breaking his dependence on others. He called me his arch nemesis with me being on the receiving end of Peter's wrath when I would get him to attempt things, like brushing his teeth, independently.

Peter not only brushed his teeth independently but also went on to live his life independently. I know he must struggle with the simpler tasks of daily life due to his physical disability but he had the determination to not let this limit or stop him.

"Hey, Peter, would you like to do a presentation to the patients on the floor?" I asked him as he left the room of a patient after giving a motivational sharing of his story to the patient and their loved one.

"I don't know. How many people?"

"About 20-25."

There was a pause before he responded.

"Just how I speak..."

Peter's speech was labored and he had the tendency of over-annunciating certain words but he was understandable.

"Whatever, I understand you loud and clear and the message you deliver is very powerful and captivates the audience. And you will be presenting with another person so you won't be alone."

I also knew Peter wanted to be a professional speaker and this would be a great starting point for him.

Over the years, my public speaking had improved but needed practice and I learned if I wasn't nervous before a speaking engagement, it would not go well. Like everything in life, practice makes perfect.

"Okay, I will do it," Peter agreed.

I met Peter before the talk and he was extremely nervous.

"Take a deep breath man," I instructed him.

"Let's go to the coffee shop on the main floor and prepare."

I was walking ahead of Peter and he followed behind me in his power wheelchair which he controlled with a joystick in one hand.

"So, how many people will be there again?" Peter asked.

I could always joke with Peter and did so when he was a patient, something he said worked well in our relationship. I don't know why I said what I was about to. Maybe I thought humor would alleviate some of his stress.

"Well, they are bussing in patients from other hospitals so 75 to 100."

When I turned back, Peter almost drove his power wheelchair into the wall. He thankfully released the joystick in time stopping before the crash.

"Woah man, was joking, about 25," I said, chuckling.

"One of these days, man," Peter said, smiling both comically and angrily.

After our prep, we returned to the floor and the dining room where patients ate. The tables were all pushed together into a huge square and around it sat patients, families, and several of my colleagues including the organizer who requested someone in a chair.

Peter's talk was breathtaking and there wasn't a dry eye in the audience. The analogies he used to describe his tribulations were original and thought-provoking and his storytelling could be best described as inspirational. I said to myself many times, 'Who is this guy?'

My eyes were always open to never underestimating persons with disabilities with what I have encountered in my life, and Peter's talk opened them even wider. I hope all would now see that there was something special in that chair.

Brothers

After Peter's unbelievable and eye-opening telling of his story to patients, I decided to approach him to do a talk with me monthly to the patients, their loved ones, and left an invite open for any therapists or students doing their clinical placements. Being a transitional hospital and with shorter length of stays, our audience would be new each month.

With Walt's, my manager at the time, permission, we got the green light to try. We would share our stories that encompassed our trials and successes with how Peter and I met, me being a therapist and him a patient. This being the link to our lecture leading to what we learned from each other that concluded our talk.

The talks were well received by all and, with the evaluation forms I handed out at the end of each talk, provided Peter and me excellent and sometimes touching feedback. I shared some of this feedback at a business meeting with my colleagues as well. Not only to share the success of our talk but also to remind some that they should not judge who they work with as their physical presentation may have been impaired but their cognition was intact.

Peter and I did the talk monthly for over two years and we spoke to over 300 patients. I made the tough decision to only do the talk quarterly. I know it was beneficial to the patients and their families and bothered me to do so but a majority of the time, I was the only one to organize.

I would set up the presentation room to accommodate wheelchairs, transport patients to and from the talk, and put things back after. I also began to realize a few therapists would sign patients up for not the patient's benefit but theirs. Our talk was 3:00pm-4:00pm and the talk would replace their therapy time, meaning an early departure from work.

I would email the therapists a week before letting them know of the talk taking place so I could enter the event in interested patients' schedules. I would also subtly plead for assistance and there were no takers. I made a point in the email to state no last-minute attendees but this also was not adhered to as the door to the presentation room would knock during the talk, with the therapist dropping off the patient and them leaving not returning to assist with transporting the patient back.

There was some push back with my decision by a higher up who knew nothing of the work involved just by me to do the talk. This was brought up at a meeting I was not even present at. This person had the rose colored glasses on not knowing that the awesome staff this higher up boasted about did not coincide with the reality of went on with preparing and carrying out my talk.

After a year, I did make the decision to do our talk every second month as I knew it benefited the patients and their families. I would be exhausted after but knew it was worth it and I also tried to live by the quote from Edmund Everrett Hale that Peter and I ended our talk with: "I am only one, but I am still one. I cannot do everything, but I can still do something."

CHAPTER TWENTY

Down the Road

After my year off at the end of 2007 and 10 months into 2008, I coped with my professional environment, initially, with some success. The ten years after however, I still struggled. Sometimes I would get bogged down as other colleagues would ignore the plight of the patients we worked with. Ignore may be too strong of a word, but that is how it felt to me.

This was why I took that year away, having gone through rehabilitation from brain injury myself and then seeing others go through it as well with less success drained me.

Why was I so fortunate? I answered this with me given a second chance to help them. What drained me and I struggled with most was when a patient's rehabilitation may have been affected by a colleague who did not put the patient first like my rehab team did.

I had to change my perseverative mindset and the several discussions with my mother over the phone helped. She knew I was wasting energy and giving too much power to the colleagues who had a negative impact on those we rehabilitated. Mom was amazing in the advice she gave me. She was empathetic of my situation knowing that it would be difficult to cope with such as it was in my face frequently. This was something I had to accept, that poor performance would have minimal to no consequences.

I had to come to the hard realization that some would end up getting the shortest straw with what therapist was assigned to them. What was even more difficult for me is that today there seemed to be more short straws than long to pick from. I was saddened, knowing that this was not just where I worked but part of society and the newer generation.

There seemed to be a lack of empathy and keeping a distance emotionally from those we supported. I know I was more sensitive due to my brain injury and having been on both sides but I met many therapists who did not go through brain injury and were empathetic and caring like me.

The one trait we did share was our age and we were from the

generation before. I caught a break having gone through rehab 20 plus years ago when that generation of therapists seemed to be the ultimate caregivers.

My journey from patient to clinician to caregiver saw the devolution of the compassionate and caring health care worker. I know it is not their fault as they are a product of their generation from a different time. A generation that focuses on what is best for them, not what is best for others. The millennial mindset was becoming more evident, something I saw everywhere not just at my job.

What frightens me is the generation to come, as one and four of us in Canada will be over 65 years of age in 2026 and will have to rely on this next generation for care.

#8

Marathon running, never thought I would run one but eight? I ran my first four for the simple reason that I could. In addition, the training got me back on track health wise.

My weight swung dramatically since my brain injury. Most people would go up and down 5-10 pounds but for me it would go up and down 30-40 in a few months span which is not good for your heart.

Weight issues and insecurity that go with them were always a battle for me from when I was teenager. I ate emotionally and after a hard day at work, a pizza and bag of chips felt deserved but this would later turn to regret. These options were also convenient as with exhaustion after work, preparing a healthy meal took time and effort. Diet and exercise were definitely instrumental to help combat my fatigue issues. When I ate healthy and was active, I felt better, carrying less weight, and then having more energy.

This was evident with my marathon training. My best time was when I weighed 168 pounds. By following a strict diet and training program, I broke the four-hour mark. I ran another marathon, finishing well over the four and a half hour mark and weighed 185 pounds. Made sense as this run felt long as I carried a 17-pound dumbbell with me as I ran.

Diet and exercise are so important for me and persons with a brain injury. I had the ability to run and be active, but others did not due to their physical disability. I would see former patients who were not active due to their disability and come back for a visit much heavier. I always respected Peter as he was very aware of his diet and appeared lean and fit even though not physically able to train as hard as me.

I decided to run an eighth and final marathon, as I was getting heavier again. I also wanted to raise money for brain injury support and research. I had done the previous three marathons to raise money for cancer research in honor of my dad and ended up raising over $3000. I wanted funds for this run to go to the provincial brain injury association and a research project I was involved with at work. Both meant a lot to me.

I sat on the board of directors for the province's brain injury association for three years and was so impressed by the support they gave persons with a brain injury and their families through advocacy, peer mentoring, and education. Fifty percent would go to help the association and their great work and the other 50 to the research department and team I worked with one day a week. Specifically to a center that was created to provide therapeutic interventions and group therapy to persons with a moderate to severe brain injury using the main technologies of the Internet and telephone. Telerehab could reach remote areas and smaller cities that did not have resources to support persons with a brain injury and their recovery.

This excited me as 22 years ago such technology was not as prevalent as today and by using these technologies, a person's rehab and recovery did not end after leaving the hospital. This could prevent chronic issues and deficits brought on by brain injury or at least minimize their affect by not only recovery but the strategies taught and learned.

I trained hard and was prepared and my fundraising efforts resulted in $3500 raised. I weighed 175 pounds going in and was not surprised by my time. #8 for Brain Injury Sake would be my last marathon but I made the lifestyle choice to continue to be active and wise with my diet choices. For my sake.

4 Hours: 19 Minutes: 58 Seconds

Above

Nine more years and I could retire early, seems so far down the road. I have to change my way of thinking to survive. I do not want to permanently wear rose-colored glasses like some and ignore what bothers me but also cannot be blind to the great work done by many.

In my lifetime involved with health care, I have encountered numerous shining stars who gave of themselves, providing the utmost care and compassion to those they supported.

From my own health care team who rehabilitated me in such a way that it gave my life direction, as I wanted to be like them and become a clinician. From the majority of nurses and doctors that tended to my father. To the numerous colleagues I have worked with and continue to work with.

I have to look to these stars to remind myself that there is good in the world and that new colleagues down the road will look as well and follow their lead.

"Hey, man."

I heard a young man speak behind me as I was talking to another patient in the hallway at work. I turned to look and when I saw the speaker, my jaw hit the floor. It was a former patient who three months earlier was discharged and when he was, I thought of the long life that lay ahead of him. Jesse was in his early 20s.

When he left rehab physically, he was progressing but at a very slow pace. He needed two people to assist him in transferring from the bed to wheelchair and was not walking. His amazing and committed physiotherapist Linda would attempt walking but needed an assistant and me to help with the walk, as she seemed to facilitate so many muscles and their movements that she looked like a puppeteer.

I would work with Jesse completing a range of motion exercises to his lower extremities to prepare his deconditioned legs for standing and walking. He was very early in his recovery and almost too acute to be with us at rehab, but that is how the system operated. A bed needed for acute care hospitals would require a person to leave earlier and if a bed became available in rehab, this would continue optimal bed flow and availability.

What I also remembered about Jesse was his loving and caring mother who was present every day during his rehab stay. We would chat and I would tell her how she reminded me of my mother when I went through rehab. I told her to not give up and with Jesse being young, he could thrive when he left rehab and that her support would be critical. At that time, I was worried I may have given false hope but knew brain injury had no time lines when it came to recovery. I was glad my hope was verified.

Jesse was very similar to me cognitively when I was early in my recovery, very flat affect with no emotions shown and seemed to be deep and almost lost in his own thoughts. I could make him laugh, which his mom appreciated. I wanted to try and normalize his life and maybe take him away from the seriousness of what was happening.

His mother gave me a beautiful gift when he was discharged with a wonderful note attached which I have taped on my computer screen at work: "Thank you for Jesse's freedom, Greg."

So, when I turned and saw this very trendy dressed, healthy young man standing in front of me with a smile, I was taken aback and stunned.

"Holy Crap, Jesse? You look amazing. How are you doing?"

"I am good. Things are going great and heading back to school in a few months."

His beautiful mother was standing behind him and seemed so proud and also thrilled at my shock. I looked at her and mouthed the word 'wow'.

I entered the gym to find Linda and saw she was working diligently with another patient, sitting beside the patient on a treatment bed.

"Linda, sorry to interrupt."

"Greg, I am really busy..." Linda knew every minute counted in a person's rehab and none could be wasted.

"You have to see and say hi to this former patient of ours. I will sit beside your patient."

She was reluctant but when she looked to the side and saw Jesse, I saw the amazement I had displayed a few minutes earlier.

"Jesse, oh my goodness. I am so proud of you."

"Thanks, Linda. You really helped me."

Jesse's mother then thanked Linda and gave her a hug. When she did, Linda held her tight and close and I could then hear sobbing and this was coming from Linda.

My heart melted as I witnessed this hug and I was so impressed by Linda. She had a caring heart and after they had left, she apologized for the crying. I told her not to apologize and to never change. This is what made her a phenomenal therapist, a star.

For the next years and beyond, I have to focus on the stars and know they will still be there in the future. I just hope they do not burn out or become rare.

What frightens me as this may be beyond health care and a societal issue. The world we live in seems to be changing daily. This includes the values of the past. How I was brought up and the work ethic I learned has changed from my grandfather, to my father, to me and now the generation after me.

All I can do is look for those stars even though they may not be able to burn as brightly due to the sky they are in.

Epilogue-19

My cell phone was vibrating as I was receiving numerous texts from my colleagues. All of the texts had the same theme: "Greg, we can get the vaccine; an email was sent out."

My heart rate began to race and I was shocked that this was happening. At the beginning of the COVID-19 pandemic, information was given that this could be our new way of life with no vaccine and if one was developed, it would take years to do so.

I went to check my work email and there was the email with a link to sign up for an appointment. I clicked on the link and the link was frozen. With a staff of over 15000 attempting all at once, this did not come as a surprise and my constant attempts did lead to great frustration.

My best friend and colleague Sophia called during my constant attempts. Sophia worked part time and is someone I worked with since I began my job 20 years ago. We would eat our lunch together, socially distanced with the window open, and talk. This kept my sanity during the pandemic.

Because of the sudden rollout, the link to access appointments continued to crash with me getting quite aggravated, with Sophia calming me down. After a couple hours, another email went out from the assistant to the CEO stating all appointments for the following day were booked and that she would send out a newer link for the next day's appointments.

I was very disappointed but very excited as for the past 10 months being immersed in COVID and wearing personal protective equipment (PPE), consisting of a facemask and a shield that covered my whole face, along with following strict protocol from hand washing, not seeing family or friends, and myself being obsessed with cleanliness and the rituals that came with this, took its toll. I had lost 30lbs in the first four weeks of the pandemic, thankfully I plateaued with my weight loss and some weight gradually returned.

I also spoke to a psychologist weekly early in the pandemic, now monthly. It was through a service work provided and from my past use of speaking to professionals I knew I would benefit. My psychologist was young and a recent graduate and all of this was new to her as no one, at least in the past 100 years, dealt with a virus that was infecting millions and killing so many.

"We will try again tomorrow. Thanks for calming me down," I stated to Sophia.

"It will happen at some point, which is exciting," Sophia replied with optimism.

I went to bed with thoughts that this nightmare possibly could come to an end. As per my usual schedule, I got up to urinate in the early morning hours and thought I would check my work email. When I checked, I went to the old link, ignoring the assistant to the CEO's email, for vaccination appointments and clicked on it. To my astonishment, over a 1000 appointments were available. I quickly typed in my information.

I would receive an appointment and was ecstatic. I would end up getting appointments for Sophia and two other of my colleagues/friends the following week as I had a day off and focused on booking theirs, albeit a very aggravating process. I did this on my off time but sadly others I worked with did not.

My one colleague had four computers going during their shift continuing to hit refresh on the link to appointments, running from one computer to the other. They were able to do this by rescheduling their patients' therapy sessions with them to the assistants and me. This colleague neglected patient care to think of themselves. This was an issue with the initial vaccine rollout as the honor system was expected to come into play.

Looking back, even I was guilty of not waiting my turn. I dealt with COVID patients not too often and worked in an environment that it was prevalent but dealt with immediately. If a patient was positive with COVID, they were isolated and we were given ample PPE to work with them. If this patient were to digress, they would be sent to an acute care hospital.

To then hear some nurses in intensive care unit (ICU) had not received their vaccination yet and were treating COVID patients with a greater chance of infection due to aerosol spread bothered me. This did not bother my colleague as they did book their appointment and boasted at the effort they put into getting it, forgetting this was at the expense of the patients they treated.

Our CEO who was amazing during the pandemic and eased my guilt by stating: "The honor system may have failed us in our initial rollout, but the most important thing is the vaccine is in the arms of people which can hopefully contain and lead to the end of the pandemic."

The same CEO five months into the pandemic, as we were in the midst of the second wave, sent me a letter of condolences as I lost my aunt, my mom's sister, to cancer. It was very heartfelt as this person, who was in charge of over 15000 employees and numerous hospitals in the midst of a once in a hundred years pandemic, took the time to send a personalized letter to me.

Reflecting on the pandemic only magnified the concerns I wrote about in ***Collateral Damage: When Caregivers No Longer Care*** and my colleagues thinking of themselves at the expense of those we rehabilitated to book their vaccination was one of too many examples of lack of care that occurred during this strenuous time when care was most needed.

The pandemic fed into my perception that some of the younger generation had a different work ethic than me, feeling entitled. This generation is also intelligent, management gave them great autonomy before the pandemic and this allowed performance issues to become embedded in our work culture.

And now that management had to deal with the protocol and processes of keeping patients, families, and workers safe from a deadly virus, no time could be spent reprimanding obvious simple issues like being on time for your patients and even seeing them. Add to the situation, no visitors were allowed into the hospital due to the potential spread of COVID, meaning no family members to advocate for their loved ones. This along with the patient population we rehabilitated having cognitive deficits and some with communication issues, therefore being unable to voice their complaints.

This created a perfect environment for some to take advantage. As my one colleague brazenly put it: "He won't know the difference of me being late or on time for his therapy" as the patient they were supposed to see had no memory or ability to orientate to time and place due to their brain injury.

I became very exhausted with everything and when I allowed a colleague and friend of mine who worked alongside of me in research to read my manuscript before the pandemic began, she stated, "Greg, you do not want to come across as just another disgruntled health care worker sharing your grievances with the world."

I was losing the fight of being able to hide my disdain and had an even shorter fuse in regard to my temper. This resulted in me being reprimanded for not being collegial with certain people whose constant neglect of patients constantly continued.

Before writing my epilogue, I did go back and try to tone down the frustration in ***Collateral Damage: When Caregivers No Longer Care*** and avoid giving the perception of the fed up employee as my research colleague and friend stated. However with the pandemic, I found that not writing and sharing my experiences with healthcare and how the industry reacted to the pandemic, it was not possible to learn how to change and prepare for not only the next pandemic but also how to make health 'uncare' less universal.

I pray the health care industry and society can change not only for me but, most importantly, also for those in need of help and care. I know one thing, if any of my family requires healthcare again, I will not be as quiet making sure to call out those who are not helping but hindering their opportunity to get better. I hope my tip sheet can be used as a resource for both the givers and receivers of care.

7 With 7: Tip Sheet to Experience And Provide Expected Care

Patient and Family

1) Research and understand what the facility you are at provides: services, hours of therapy, length of stay. Inform yourself early as to the next steps following hospitalization so that you fully understand services available to you following discharge. Keep a journal throughout the hospitalization process and following discharge. Make note of your milestones in the journal having a comparison to look back and see your progress. On those discouraging days, when you are feeling stuck, it is really helpful to look back over the journal to be able to self-correct and say, hey, look where you were a month or six months ago and look where you are now.
2) Get to know your circle of care team; ask questions about their training and the techniques they use. This will make the team aware you are interested and invested in the process making clinicians more accountable knowing you are observant and informed. Ask all staff interacting with you or family member their name, even if a short interaction. Look at name badges. Make it known you are taking note of anyone you or your family member interacts with.
3) Put pictures up of your loved ones within room. Make health care workers see "you" not your diagnosis or injury. Remember the phrase "squeaky wheel gets the oil" is true. Don't be afraid to speak up/advocate and give feedback to those you feel are not meeting your or your loved ones' needs. Deliver feedback in a way that is respectful, remembering they are trying to help.
4) Where possible, attend therapy sessions, appointments, and information sessions with family members to enhance your learning along with information seeking to better prepare for the future and what may lie ahead. Be positive and understanding within reason. The hospital environment is busy, clinicians are overworked.
5) Document and track activities, conversations, and therapies to confirm concerns that arise and for constructive feedback. If possible, have witnesses. Talk to the relevant team member of your concerns. Try not to over-explain when voicing your concern – be to the point, clear. If it continues, take the next step to be heard, speak

with the Unit Manager and/or contact Patient Relations. Request a chart review. Sadly, if needed, go public. This will make a difference for not only you but also those in the future, preventing possible harm or substandard care from happening again.

6) Complete any facility questionnaires regarding impressions and delivery of care. It may not make a difference for you or your family, but it will for another patient and could make all the difference.
7) Families please seek caregiver support. You play a crucial role in the success of a discharge plan. Caregivers need to maintain strength and ability for the longer term and provide a voice for those without one.

Clinicians and Management

1) Always follow the Golden Rule: treat others how you or your loved ones would like to be treated.
2) Pause and remember that patient challenges are due to their brain injury, ailment and current situation and may not be purposeful. We are dealing with patients and caregivers sometimes at their most vulnerable state who are dealing with tremendous loss. Are your relationships with patients based on the mindset of "power-with" vs. "power over"? Am I aware of the power-differential that exists between myself and my patients? Am I looking at my interactions with this in mind?
3) Speak up and advocate for those patients who do not have a voice or support. Are you seeing a patient as a whole person or just as a label, number, or diagnosis?
4) Listen to the patients you serve. Do not be afraid to give constructive feedback to those who can improve upon their professionalism and meet facility standards/expectations. By doing so, this opens up communication that can lead to solving the issue.
5) Be a collective when addressing ongoing performance issues. This will make dealing with the issue easier and that it is not personal and the colleague does not feel targeted specifically by you.
6) Managers: track and document performance issues to solve them. This will create work for you but is for the patient's best interest and care. By doing so, this type of performance does not become tolerated and embedded. This results in creating a culture of providing expected care.
7) Take care of self first so that you can be your best with patients and families. Staff need to recognize they are burned out and seek the appropriate support.

Index

CPSIA information can be obtained
at www.ICGtesting.com
Printed in the USA
BVHW041937070822
643772BV00005B/8

9 781913 976187